Contents

Preface to Fourth Edition

Throughout the last editions we have endeavoured gradually to remove the more academic information and include data we consider to be more clinically useful. This development has continued, using suggestions from many sources. We have made the information more accessible and have updated it to conform with changing medical practice. The critical care section is new and includes the Glasgow coma score and APACHE II score to encourage the critical auditing of clinical performance that is becoming increasingly necessary these days. Thirty-seven informative colour diagrams have been added to the anaesthesia section. The more logical format and greatly enlarged index should make information retrieval significantly easier.

As usual, many clinicians have helped us with their particular expertise, and we would particularly like to thank Guys Hospital Poisons Centre, Dr Ron Hill, Dr Jim Johnstone, Dr Martin Rothman and Dr Brian Colvin as well as many others who have made a contribution. The colour section was kindly provided by Astra Pharmaceuticals Ltd.

We would appreciate any comments from our colleagues who use and read this book about any errors or ommissions that may have crept into this edition; we hope they are few and of a minor nature.

Finally, our thanks to the staff of Blackwell Scientific Publications who have, as usual, provided tolerant guidance throughout the preparation of this edition.

R. P. H. Dunnill
M. P. Colvin

Clinical and Resuscitative Data

A Compendium of Intensive, Medical and Anaesthetic Resuscitative Data

R. P. H. DUNNILL

MBBS FFARCS
Consultant Anaesthetist
Bournemouth and Poole Hospitals

M. P. COLVIN

BSc MBBS FFARCS
Consultant Anaesthetist
The London Hospital

FOURTH EDITION

Blackwell Scientific Publications

OXFORD LONDON EDINBURGH

BOSTON MELBOURNE

© 1977, 1979, 1984, 1989 by
Blackwell Scientific Publications
Editorial offices:
Osney Mead, Oxford OX2 0EL
   (*Orders*: Tel. 0865 240201)
8 John Street, London WC1N 2ES
23 Ainslie Place, Edinburgh EH3 6AJ
3 Cambridge Center, Suite 208
   Cambridge, Massachusetts 02142, USA
107 Barry Street, Carlton
   Victoria 3053, Australia

First published 1977
Second edition 1979
German edition 1983
Third edition 1984
Fourth edition 1989

Set by Macmillan India Ltd,
Bangalore 25
Printed and bound in Great Britain by
Butler & Tanner Ltd, Frome and London

DISTRIBUTORS

USA
   Year Book Medical Publishers
   200 North LaSalle Street
   Chicago, Illinois 60601
   (*Orders*: Tel. (312) 726-9733)

Canada
   The C. V. Mosby Company
   5240 Finch Avenue East
   Scarborough, Ontario
   (*Orders*: Tel. (416) 298-1588)

Australia
   Blackwell Scientific Publications
   (Australia) Pty Ltd
   107 Barry Street
   Carlton, Victoria 3053
   (*Orders*: Tel. (03) 347-0300)

British Library
Cataloguing in Publication Data

Dunnill, R. P. H. (Richard Paul Hyde)
   Clinical and resuscitative data—4th ed.
   1. Man. Resuscitation: Technical data
   I. Title   II. Colvin, M. P. (Michael Peter)
   615.8'043

   ISBN 0-632-02407-0

Preface to First Edition

In practical and emergency situations there is often an urgent need for numerical data, formulae and general guidelines for treatment. It has been our purpose to provide this information in a logical and easy-to-find manner. This book is in no way a textbook or even a book on how to treat patients, it is a compendium of that data which is often hard to find but needed quickly in resuscitation procedures.

It is intended for all grades of junior staff in most specialities, especially those involved in accident and emergency departments, intensive care and other resuscitation areas.

The data come from numerous sources and we have tried to include facts and formulae that will be safe to use and acceptable to most schools of thought. The book is arranged in sections and subsections, as shown in the list of contents. References are given at the foot of subsections and space is provided for personal notes and additions as new information and drugs come on to the market.

Whilst every effort has been made to ensure the accuracy of the information given, the authors would be grateful for any corrections as well as ideas for further inclusions.

We have in all cases endeavoured to trace and acknowledge the original source of material used. In addition we would like to thank the following for their kind help in producing this book: Dr Volans and Robin Braithwaite of Guy's Hospital, National Poisons Centre; Dr Sterndale, Consultant Haematologist; Mr Hoskins, Chief Pharmacist; Mr Stockhill, Chief Technician, Biochemistry Department; Mr D. Rodgers, Department of Medical Illustration, all at the Kent and Canterbury Hospital; Professor Strunin, Dr Ainley Walker, Dr Potter, Dr Wedley, for correcting the proofs; Mrs J. Atterbury and Mrs M. Allen for their secretarial help; and last but by no means least Blackwell Scientific Publications for their help and encouragement.

R. P. H. Dunnill
B. E. Crawley

Abbreviations

<	less than	DIC	disseminated intravascular coagulation
>	greater than	DVT	deep vein thrombosis
♀	female	EACA	ε-aminocaproic acid
♂	male	ECF	extracellular fluid
ABG	arterial blood gases	ECG	electrocardiogram
AF	atrial fibrillation	ECM	external cardiac massage
alb.	albumin	ESR	erythrocyte sedimentation rate
alt die	alternate days	FDP	fibrin degradation products
APS	acute physiological score		
ATN	acute tubular necrosis	FEV	forced expiratory volume
ATPS	ambient temperature and pressure saturated with water vapour	FFP	fresh frozen plasma
		FiO_2	fractional concentration of inspired oxygen
AV	atrioventricular	ft	feet
B	bolus dose	g	grams
b.d.	*bis die* (twice a day)	GA	general anaesthetic
BM	blood sugar test strips	GCS	Glasgow coma scale
BP	blood pressure	GI	gastrointestinal
BSA	body surface area	h	hour(s)/hourly
BSP	bromsulphthalein	H^+	hydrogen ion
BTPS	body temperature and pressure saturated with water vapour	HBCO	carboxyhaemoglobin
		HCT	haematocrit
		HIV	human immunosuppressive virus
Ca	calcium		
cal	calories	H_2O	water
CHO	carbohydrate	HPPF	human plasma protein fraction
Cl	chloride ion		
CNS	central nervous system	I	infusion
CO	carbon monoxide	ICD	isocitric dehydrogenase
CO	cardiac output	i.m.	intramuscular
CSF	cerebrospinal fluid	INR	International Normalized Ratio
CVA	cerebrovascular accident		
CVP	central venous pressure	ITP	idiopathic thrombo-cytopaenic purpura
D	daily		
D/min	drops per minute	ITU	intensive therapy unit
DC	direct current	iu	international units
DD	divided doses	i.v.	intravenously
DDAVP	deamino-D-arginine vasopressin		

J	joules	NSAID	non-steroidal anti-inflammatory drug
K	kelvin		
K$^+$	potassium ion	o	orally
KA units	King–Armstrong units	PABA	para-aminobenzoic acid
KCCT	kaolin cephalin clotting time	PAWP	pulmonary artery wedge pressure
kg	kilograms	Pco_2	partial pressure carbon dioxide
kPa	kilopascals		
l	litre	PCV	packed cell volume
lb	pound weight	percut.	percutaneously
lb F/in^2	pounds force per square inch	pH	hydrogen ion concentration
LDH	lactic dehydrogenase	PIG	potassium insulin glucose regime
LFT	liver function tests		
μ	micro (0.001 of milli)	Po_2	partial pressure oxygen
μg	micrograms	PO$_4$	phosphate
M	molar	PPF	plasma protein fraction
MAOI	monoamine oxidase inhibitor	PR	P to R wave interval on the ECG
MCHC	mean corpuscular haemoglobin concentration	p.r.n.	take when necessary
		PT	prothrombin time
		PTI	prothrombin index
MCV	mean corpuscular volume	PTR	prothrombin ratio
mEq/l	milliequivalents per litre	PTT	partial thromboplastin time
Mg	magnesium		
min	minutes	q.d.s.	quater die sumendum (four times daily)
min vol	minute volume		
ml	millilitres	QRS	ventricular complex on the ECG
mm	millimetres		
mmHg	millimetres of mercury	QT	Q to T wave interval on the ECG
mmol	millimoles		
Mn	manganese	RBBB	right bundle branch block
mol wt	molecular weight	RBC	red blood cell count
mosmol	milliosmoles	rect.	rectally
MSU	midstream specimen of urine	RQ	respiratory quotient
		RSR	R to S to R wave of the ECG
N	newtons		
N$_2$	nitrogen	s	seconds
Na	sodium	sat.	saturation
NaCl	sodium chloride	s.c.	subcutaneously
NaHCO$_3$	sodium bicarbonate	SGOT	serum glutamic oxalic transaminase
NG	nasogastric		
NH$_4$	ammonia	SGPT	serum glutamic pyruvic transaminase
nmol	nanomoles		
nocte	take at night	SI units	International System of Units
NPH	neutral protamine hagedorn (insulin)		
		ST	S to T wave on the ECG
N/S	0.9% normal saline solution		
		stat.	immediately

STPD	standard temperature and pressure dry	u	unit
subling.	take sublingually	VC	vital capacity
SWG	standard wire gauge	VF	ventricular fibrillation
tab	tablet	VMA	vanillylmandelic acid
TCT	thrombin clotting time	vol.	volume
t.d.s.	three times daily dose	VT	ventricular tachycardia
TIBC	total iron binding capacity	W	watt
TPN	total parenteral nutrition	WBC	white blood cell count
TSH	thyroid-stimulating hormone	wt	weight
TT	thrombin time	yr	year
		Zn	zinc

Section 1
Acid Base Balance

1.1 pH conversion to H$^+$ nanomoles

pH units	H$^+$ nmol	pH units	H$^+$ nmol
3	1000 000	6	1000
3.1	794 200	6.1	794.2
3.2	630 900	6.2	630.9
3.3	501 200	6.3	501.2
3.4	398 100	6.4	398.1
3.5	316 300	6.5	316.3
3.6	251 200	6.6	251.2
3.7	199 500	6.7	199.5
3.8	158 500	6.8	158.5
3.9	125 900	6.9	125.9
4	100 100	7	100
4.1	79 420	7.1	79.42
4.2	63 090	7.2	63.09
4.3	50 120	7.3	50.12
4.4	39 810	7.4	39.81
4.5	31 630	7.5	31.63
4.6	25 120	7.6	25.12
4.7	19 950	7.7	19.95
4.8	15 850	7.8	15.85
4.9	12 590	7.9	12.59
5	10 000	8	10
5.1	7942	8.1	7.942
5.2	6309	8.2	6.309
5.3	5012	8.3	5.012
5.4	3981	8.4	3.981
5.5	3163	8.5	3.163
5.6	2512	8.6	2.512
5.7	1995	8.7	1.995
5.8	1585	8.8	1.585
5.9	1259	8.9	1.259
6	1000	9	1

1.2 Acid base correction formulae

1.2.1 Correction of metabolic acidosis

Give base deficit × $\frac{1}{3}$ weight in kg ($\frac{1}{5}$ weight is more accurate in adults) as mmol sodium bicarbonate.

1.2.2 Correction of metabolic alkalosis in adults

Give either:
250 mg Diamox 6 hourly until urine pH > 7 (2–6 hour delay before full effect). Maintain K^+ 4.5–5 mmol/l to improve effect
or:
Ammonium chloride 2 g t.d.s. orally.

As the pH falls by 0.1 unit the K^+ in plasma rises 0.6 mmol approx. and vice versa.

1.2.3 To correct hyperkalaemia in adults

Give either:
20 units of soluble insulin with 30 g of glucose
or:
Na^+ Resonium or Ca^{++} Resonium 15 g t.d.s. orally or rectally.

2

Section 2
**Anaesthesia:
General and Local**

2

2.1 Physical properties of anaesthetic gases and vapours

Name	BP (°C)	Mol wt	Specific gravity Gas	Specific gravity Liquid	SVP at 20°C (mmHg)	AD95 (%)	MAC (%)	Ostwald solubility coefficient 37°C — Oil/H_2O	Blood/gas	H_2O	Flamm. O_2 (%)
Carbon dioxide	−79	44	1.98	1.20	42 280					55.5	0
Chloroform	61	119	4.10	1.47	160	10	0.5	100	10	40	0
Cyclopropane	−34	42	1.45	0.58	4800		9.2	34	0.46	0.20	2–60
Divinyl ether	28	70	2.42	0.78	560		3	41	2.6	1.40	2–85
Enflurane	57	184	7.54	1.50	180	1.9	1.7	120	1.9	0.78	4–100
Ether	35	74	2.56	0.72	425	2.2	1.9	3.2	12.0	13	2–82
Ethyl chloride	13	65	2.23	0.90	988		2	75	3	1.2	4–67
Ethylene	−104	28	0.97	0.34			65	1.3	0.14	0.09	3–80
Fluoroxene	43	126	4.40	1.10	290	75	3.5	94	1.4	0.85	4–100
Halothane	50	197	6.80	1.90	243	0.9	0.8	220	2.5	0.80	0
Helium	−269	4	0.18	0.13							0
Isoflurane	49	185	7.54	1.51	250	1.6	1.2	120	1.4	0.62	6–100
Methoxyflurane	105	165	5.70	1.40	25	0.2	0.2	400	13	4.50	5–28
Nitrogen	−196	28	1.25	0.80						1.20	0
Nitrous oxide	−89	44	1.53	1.87	39 760	110	105	2.2	0.47	0.44	0
Oxygen	−183	32	1.10	1.14						2.40	0
Trichlorethylene	87	131	4.40	1.47	60	0.4	0.3	400	9	1.70	9–65

BP = boiling point; SVP = saturated vapour pressure. AD95 = approaches to the theoretical minimum anaesthetic concentration by estimating the dose that anaesthetizes 95% of the population. MAC = minimum alveolar concentration (the concentration of anaesthetic agent required to produce lack of reflex response to a skin incision in 50% of subjects).
Specific gravity = relative density of the fluid to that of water (liquid) or in the case of a vapour to that of dry air (gases)

2.2 Pressure and contents of gases in anaesthesia and medicine

2.2.1 Medical gas cylinder data

Gas	Colour code UK Top	UK Body	USA Top	USA Body	International standard Top	International standard Body	Critical Temp. (°C)	Critical Press. (bar)	Fill press (bar)	B	C	D	E	F	G	H
Oxygen	White	Black	Green	Black	White		−119	50.8	137		170	340	680	1360	3400	6800
Nitrous oxide	Blue	Blue	Blue	Blue	Blue		36.5	71.7	50			450	900	1800	3600	9000
Entonox	White Blue	Blue							137			500		2000	5000	
Air	White Black	Grey	Yellow	Grey	Black	White	−141	37	137				640	1280	3200	6400
Carbon dioxide	Grey		Grey		Grey		31	72.8	50		450		1800			

Cylinder sizes (litres)

2

Carbon dioxide/ oxygen	Grey White	Black	Grey	Green	Grey	White			137			1360 3400
Helium	Brown		Brown	Brown	Brown		−268	2.26	137		300	1200
Helium/ oxygen	White/ brown	Black	Yellow	Brown	Brown	White			137		600	1200
Cyclopropane	Orange		Orange		Orange		125	54	5	180		

Empty cylinder weight (kg)	1.6	2	3.4	5.4	14.5	34.5	68.9
Cylinder dimensions (mm)	330 × 76	430 × 89	535 × 102	865 × 102	930 × 140	1320 × 178	1520 × 229

* *Critical temperature* = temperature to which a gas must cool before it will liquefy under pressure

† *Critical pressure* = pressure required to liquefy a gas at its critical temperature

2.3 Anaesthetic endotracheal tube and circuit data

2.3.1 Endotracheal tube size

	Tube size				Tracheostomy			
		Int. diam.	Length (cm)		Int.	French	Ext.	Broncho-
Age (years)	Magill	(mm)	Oral	Nasal	(mm)	gauge	(mm)	scope
0–3 months	00	3	10					⎱ Suckling
	0A	3.5	10–11					⎰
3–6 months	0	4	12	15	4		5.5	⎱ Infant
6–12 months	1	4.5	12	15	4.5		6	⎰
2	2	5	13	16	5	21	7	⎫
3	2	5	13	16	5	21		⎪
4	3	5.5	14	17	5.5	24		⎬ Child
5	3	5.5	14	17	5.5	24		⎪
6	4	6	15	18	6	27	8	⎭
7	4	6	15	18	6	27		⎫
8	5	6.5	16	19	6.5	28	8.5	⎬ Adolescent
9	5	6.5	16	19	6.5	29		⎪
10	6	7	17	20	7	30	9	⎭
11	6	7	17	20	7	30	9	⎱ Small
12	7	7.5	18	21	7.5	32	10	⎰ adult
13	7	7.5	18	21	7.5	32	10	⎫
14	8	8	21	24	8	33	11	⎪
15	8	8	21	24	8	33		⎪
16	8	8	21	24	8	33		⎬ Large
17	9	9	22	25	9	36	12	⎪ adult
18	9	9	22	25	9	36		⎪
20	10	9.5	23	26	10	39	13	⎪
22	10+	10+	23	26	11+	42	14	⎭

Below 8–10 years, non-cuffed tubes should be used.

2.3.2 Endotracheal tube size formulae

The following formulae give rule of thumb methods of assessing tube size, tube lengths, etc., with an accuracy of $\pm 10\%$.

1 Tube size $= \dfrac{\text{Age (yr)}}{4} + 4.5$ mm.

2 Oral length $= 12 + \dfrac{\text{Age (yr)}}{2}$ cm.

3 Nasal length = $15 + \dfrac{\text{Age (yr)}}{2}$ cm.

4 Dead space = 2 ml/kg or 1 ml/lb.

5 Tidal volume = 3 × dead space or 7–10 ml/kg above 10 kg weight.

2

2.4 Drugs in anaesthesia

2.4.1 Premedication in children

It is usual to give anaesthetic drugs to children according to their body weight. The paediatric prescribing regimen from the section on drugs is also repeated here as another rough guide to drug doses in children.

Paediatric prescribing regimen

Age	Average wt (kg)	Proportion of adult dose (%)
2 months	3.2	10
4 months	6.5	15
1 year	10	25
5 years	18	33
7 years	23	50
12 years	37	75
15 years	55	85
Adult	66	100

Anticholinergic drugs orally or i.m.

Weight (kg)	Atropine (mg)	Hyoscine (mg)	Glycopyrrolate (mg)
0–12	0.2	0.15	0.1
12–20	0.3	0.2	0.15
20–50	0.4	0.3	0.2
>50	0.6	0.4	0.4

Sedative and analgesic drugs

Drug	Dose	Route
Vallergan Forte	2 4 mg/kg	o
Omnopon	0.3 mg/kg	i.m.
Pethidine	1 mg/kg	i.m.
Phenergan	0.4 mg/kg	i.m.

These drugs are those most commonly used in children. Doses of other drugs are shown in Section 2.4.2, p. 13.

2.4.2 Drugs used by infusion for analgesia and sedation in intensive care and anaesthesia

All these drugs, grouped here according to their basic action, can be used either alone or in combination as an infusion, to provide variable degrees of analgesia, sedation or anaesthesia in the intensive therapy unit.

These powerful drugs must only be administered by drip counter or infusion pump under *close* supervision by nursing and medical staff who fully understand their pharmacology. They should not be used outside an intensive therapy or high dependency unit or an operating theatre.

The figures suggested are only basic guidelines; wide variations in dose may be necessary in clinical practice, requiring rapid adjustment initially to achieve the effect required, particularly for full surgical anaesthesia. These variations are due to:

1 Variation in individual patient response.

2 The purpose of the infusion, ranging from analgesia, through sedation to full surgical anaesthesia, which would require much higher doses than the figures quoted here.

3 Drug combinations: for instance, the dose of midazolam required for sedation will be reduced by a simultaneous infusion of an analgesic like pethidine or fentanyl.

Optimal, reversible sedation can only be achieved by constant reassessment and vigilance.

Drugs	µg/kg/min	mg/h (70 kg)
Anaesthetics and sedatives		
Chlormethiazole (Heminevrin) 0.8%	114–457	480–1920
Methohexitone (Brietal) 1%	60	252
Midazolam (Hypnovel) 0.5%	0.6–2.4	2.5–10
Propofol (Diprivan) 1%	24–48	100–200
Thiopentone 2.5%	60	250
Analgesics		
Alfentanil (Rapifen) 0.05%	0.5–1	2.1–4.2
Papaveretum (Omnopon)	1.2	5
Pethidine	2.4–12	10–50
Fentanyl (Sublimaze)	0.06	0.25
Muscle relaxants		
Atracurium (Tracrium)	5–10	21–42
Vecuronium (Norcuron)	0.8–1.3	3.5–5.6
Benzodiazepine antagonist		
Flumazenil	0.02–0.1	0.1–0.4

2.4.3 Premedication and general anaesthetic drugs and doses

Non-proprietary name	Adult dose	Paediatric dose
Anaesthetic induction drugs		
Etomidate	20 mg i.v.	0.3 mg/kg
Ketamine	500 mg i.m.	8 mg/kg i.m.
	150 mg i.v.	2 mg/kg i.v.
Methohexitone	100 mg i.v.	1.5 mg/kg
Propofol	2–2.5 mg/kg i.v.	
	6–12 mg/kg/h infusion	
Thiopentone	300 mg i.v.	4.5 mg/kg
Analgesics		
Alfentanil	0.25–1 mg i.v.	15–50 µg/kg i.v.
Buprenorphine	0.2–0.4 mg subling.	
	0.3–0.6 mg i.m.	Not in children
Diamorphine	5 mg o., i.m., i.v.	
	Extradural: 2–5 mg in 10 ml saline	
Fentanyl	50–100 µg i.m.	1–3 µg/kg i.v.
	50–250 µg i.v.	
Fentanyl 50 µg/ml + Droperidol 2.5 µg/ml	1–2 ml i.m.	0.4–1.5 ml i.m. for premed.
	Induction: 6–8 ml	
	Maintain: 1–2 ml	

Non-proprietary name	Adult dose	Paediatric dose
Meptazinol	200 mg 3–6 h o 75–100 mg 2–4 h i.m. 50–100 mg i.v.	
Methadone	5–10 mg o, i.m., i.v.	

Morphine	10–15 mg i.m.,
	5 mg i.v.
	Extradural and intrathecal:
	  2–4 mg preservative free
	  morphine in 10 ml saline
		0.2 mg/kg i.m.
		0.1 mg/kg i.v.

Papaveretum	20 mg i.m. 4 h 2.5 mg i.v.	0.4 mg/kg i.m.
Pentazocine	30–60 mg s.c., i.m., i.v.	Max. 1 mg/kg i.m. 0.5 mg/kg i.v.
Pethidine	50 mg 4 h o 50–100 mg i.m. 4 h 10–20 mg i.v. 50–150 mg 4 h o	6–12 yr: 25 mg 4 h o 1 mg/kg i.m. 4 h 0.5–2 mg/kg o
Phenoperidine	1–2 mg i.v.	0.1–0.15 mg/kg i.v.

Doses of other analgesic drugs can be found in Section 11, p. 171

Anticholinergic drugs

Atropine	Premed 0.6 mg i.m. Reversal of relaxants 1–2 mg i.v.	See Section 2.4.1 0.02 mg/kg i.v.
Glycopyrrolate	0.2–0.4 mg i.m., i.v.	0.004–0.008 mg/kg i.m., i.v.
	Relaxant reversal: adults and children 0.01 mg/kg with 0.05 mg/kg neostigmine	
Hyoscine	0.4 mg i.m.	See Section 2.4.1
Propantheline	30 mg i.v.	

Anticholinesterase drugs

Neostigmine	2.5 mg i.v.	0.05 mg/kg

Antiemetic drugs

Cyclizine	50 mg t.d.s. o 50 mg i.m., i.v.	1–10 yr 25 mg t.d.s. o
Droperidol	5 mg i.m.	0.3 mg/kg i.m.
Metoclopramide	5–10 mg o, i.m., i.v.	1 yr: 1 mg o, i.m., i.v. 3–5 yr: 2 mg 6–14 yr: 2.5 mg
Perphenazine	4 mg t.d.s. o 5 mg i.m. 6 h	Not in children
Prochlorperazine	12.5 mg i.m.	
Thiethylperazine	10 mg t.d.s. o 6.5 mg i.m. 6.5 mg rectally	Not in children

Non-proprietary name	Adult dose	Paediatric dose
Benzodiazepine reversal		
Flumazenil	200 μg i.v. repeat 100 μg at 15 s interval up to 500 μg Max. dose 2 mg 100–400 μg/h infusion	
Drugs in deliberate hypotension		
Diazoxide	300 mg i.v. rapidly	5 mg/kg i.v.
Glyceryl trinitrate	50 mg in 50 ml 4 ml/h starting dose or 67 μg/min	
Hydralazine	20 mg i.v. slowly	
Labetalol	10–20 mg i.v. Repeat depending on effect, or infusion 1 mg/ml	
Nitroprusside	50 mg in 500 ml 5% dextrose Max. 400 μg/min. Use drip counter and burette	
Pentolinium	Up to 10 mg in 0.5 mg increments	
Phentolamine	Up to 10 mg i.v. in 1 mg increments Infusion: 10 mg in 100 ml; adjust rate for effect	
Trimetaphan	250 mg in 500 ml 5% dextrose Infuse according to response	
Muscle relaxant drugs		
(a) Depolarizing		
Suxamethonium bromide or chloride	75–100 mg i.v.	1 mg/kg
(b) Non-depolarizing (for children under 6 months half the paediatric dose should be used)		
Alcuronium	15–20 mg i.v.	0.25 mg/kg
Atracurium	0.3–0.6 mg/kg	0.3–0.6 mg/kg
Gallamine	120 mg i.v.	1.5 mg/kg
Pancuronium	6 mg i.v.	0.07 mg/kg
Tubocurarine	35 mg i.v.	0.4 mg/kg
Vecuronium	0.08–0.1 mg/kg	Not in children
Narcotic antagonists		
Naloxone	0.1–0.2 mg i.m. i.v.	1.5–3 μg/kg neonates: 0.01 mg/kg
Sedatives and premedicants		
Amylobarbitone	200 mg o	
Chloral hydrate	1–2 g o	30–50 mg/kg o

Non-proprietary name	Adult dose	Paediatric dose
Chlorpromazine	25–50 mg o	Over 5 yr. $\frac{1}{3}$–$\frac{1}{2}$
	25–50 mg i.m.	Adult dose o, i.m.
	5–10 mg i.v.	Under 5 yr. 5–10 mg o, i.m.
Diazepam	5–10 mg o, i.m., i.v.	0.1 mg/kg
Droperidol	5–10 mg i.m., i.v.	0.2–0.3 mg/kg i.v.
	5–20 mg o	0.3–0.6 mg/kg i.m.
		0.2–0.6 mg/kg o
Haloperidol	5 mg i.m., o	
Lorazepam	2–4 mg o	
	0.025–0.5 mg/kg i.m., i.v.	Not in children
Midazolam	0.07 mg/kg i.v., i.m.	
Pentobarbitone	100–200 mg o	Not in children
Promazine	50 mg i.m.	Proportional to adult
	25–100 mg o	dose on weight basis
Promethazine	25–50 mg o, i.m.	
Quinalbarbitone	200–300 mg o	50–100 mg o
Temazepam	10–30 mg o	
Trimeprazine	3–4.5 mg/kg o	2–4 mg/kg o
Vasoconstrictor drugs		
Ephedrine	Up to 10 mg i.v.	
	10–30 mg i.m.	
Metaraminol	1 mg i.v., 5 mg i.m.	
Methoxamine	5 mg i.m., i.v.	

2.4.4 Treatment of malignant hyperpyrexia

This condition, which occurs in susceptible individuals exposed to a precipitating drug, is characterized by a rapid rise in temperature to very high levels during general anaesthesia. There may be a family history of death during anaesthesia.

Signs and symptoms
Rapid rise in temperature
Muscle rigidity
Tachycardia
Tachypnoea
Cyanosis
Dysrhythmia
Myoglobinuria
Acute renal failure
Failure of coagulation

2

Laboratory findings

Hyperkalaemia
Hypoxia
Hypercarbia
Hyperphosphataemia
Hypocalcaemia
Clotting screen may demonstrate disseminated intravascular coagulation (DIC).

Treatment

As soon as this condition is suspected:
1 Discontinue anaesthesia and surgery.
2 Inflate lungs with 100% oxygen through a clean circuit.
3 Start surface cooling.
4 Give dantrolene 1 mg/kg i.v. at 5–10 min intervals to a total of 10 mg/kg.
5 Correct potassium with glucose and insulin intravenously.
6 Give methyl prednisolone 30 mg/kg.
7 Correct acidosis with sodium bicarbonate.
8 Give an initial dose of mannitol 20%, 20 g or 100 ml.
9 If DIC develops, consult a haematologist.

Possible precipitating factors

1 Inhalation agents: halothane, enflurane, fluoroxene, methoxyflurane, trichloroethylene, diethyl ether, chloroform, cyclopropane, isoflurane.
2 Non-depolarizing muscle relaxants: tubocurarine, gallamine.
3 Depolarizing muscle relaxant: suxamethonium.

Probable safe drugs

Regional blockade
Thiopentone, althesin, ketamine
Nitrous oxide
Pancuronium
Fentanyl
Droperidol
Promethazine
Propofol

2.4.5 Antacids in obstetric anaesthesia

Obstetric patients undergoing elective or emergency procedures, whether in labour or not, should be protected as far as possible from the dangers of inhalation of stomach contents. An attempt should be made to reduce the volume of stomach contents and increase their pH above 2.5.

There is evidence that magnesium trisilicate may itself cause lung damage, and the following regimen is suggested.

Patients in labour

Oral administration of 0.3 molar sodium citrate 30 ml, 15 minutes before anaesthesia.

If labour has been particularly prolonged, and the patient has received pethidine, consideration should be given to emptying the stomach and giving sodium citrate before induction of anaesthesia.

Elective obstetric procedures

Cimetidine 400 mg orally *nocte* and cimetidine 400 mg i.m. 90 minutes before anaesthesia. Sodium citrate 30 ml can also be given 15 minutes before anaesthesia.

2.5 Local anaesthetics

2.5.1 Local anaesthetic drugs and doses

Pharmacological (and proprietary) name	Amount supplied (%)	Max. adult dose without adrenaline (mg)	Onset time (min)	Duration (h)	Spinal solution	Epidural solution (%)
Bupivacaine (Marcain)	0.25–0.5	150	15–45	3–6	2 ml 0.5%	0.25–0.5
Bupivacaine (heavy)	0.5	150	10–20	2–4	3 ml 0.5%	—
Cinchocaine (Nupercaine)	0.02–0.1	75	5–15	3–4	4 ml 0.5%	—
Cocaine	4–10	100 (topical only)				
Etidocaine (Duranest)	0.5–1	300	6–10	5–7	—	1
Lignocaine (heavy)	5	200	5–10	1–1½	1–2 ml	—
Lignocaine (Xylocaine)	0.5–1.5	150–200	5–15	1.25–3	4 ml 4%	1–2
Mepivacaine (Carbocaine)	0.5–2	200–300	5–15	1.25–3	2 ml 4%	1–2
Prilocaine (Citanest)	1–2	400–600	5–15	3–5	2 ml 4%	1–2
Procaine (Novocaine)	0.5–2	700–1000	5–15	0.75–1.5	4 ml 5%	2
Tetracaine/amethocaine (Pontocaine)	0.05–0.25	150–200	15–45	3.5–6	2 ml 1%	0.25

2

Toxic side effects of local anaesthetics
1 Cardiac:
myocardial depression
bradycardia

2 Central nervous system:
excitation—convulsion
inhibition—coma

3 Anaphylaxis:
rash
hypotension
bronchospasm

Treatment of side effects
1 Cardiac:
atropine 0.6 mg
isoprenaline 4 μg i.v. (see Section 6.5, p. 119)
oxygen

2 Central nervous system:
anticonvulsants, diazepam 10–20 mg i.v.
intubation and ventilation
fluids
oxygen

3 Anaphylaxis:
aminophylline 250 mg i.v.
adrenaline 0.5 mg s.c.
fluids
intubation and ventilation
oxygen
hydrocortisone 200 mg i.v.

2.5.2 Dermatomes: the whole body

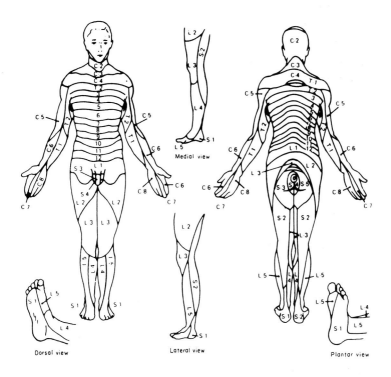

Dermatomes of the body representing segmental distribution of spinal nerves according to classical teachings, based on Foerster's data.

2.5.3 Dermatomes: the limbs

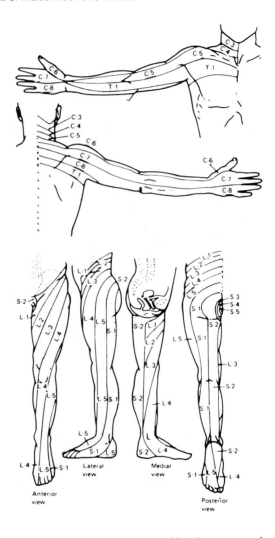

Dermatomes of the limbs as determined by the pattern of
hypoalgesia from loss of a single nerve root.

2.5.4 Sclerotomes

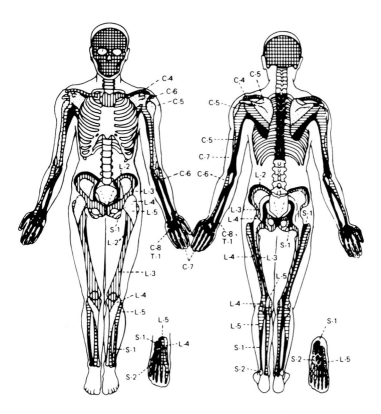

The various patterns moderate the fields of supply of each spinal segment. The skull is innervated by the trigeminal nerve and posterior primary rami of C2; the vertebrae by the posterior divisions of the respective spinal nerves, and the ribs by both posterior and anterior primary divisions of the respective spinal nerves. The insets show the sclerotomes of the feet.

2.5.5 Male genitourinary nerve supply

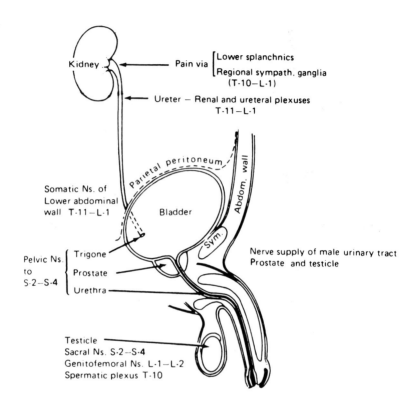

Kidney

Pain via ⎡Lower splanchnics
        ⎣Regional sympath. ganglia
        (T-10—L-1)

Ureter — Renal and ureteral plexuses
        T-11—L-1

Parietal peritoneum

Abdom. wall

Somatic Ns. of
Lower abdominal
wall T-11—L-1

Bladder

Sym.

Nerve supply of male urinary tract
Prostate and testicle

Pelvic Ns. ⎧Trigone
to   ⎨Prostate
S-2—S-4   ⎩Urethra

Testicle
Sacral Ns. S-2—S-4
Genitofemoral Ns. L-1—L-2
Spermatic plexus T-10

2.5.6 Female genitourinary nerve supply

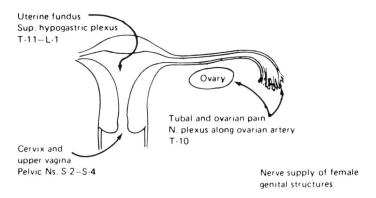

Nerve supply of female
genital structures

2.5.7 Other types of block and local anaesthetic doses

This is not a text on technique, merely a dose reminder. The total dose is given when two or more injections are required to complete the block.

Block	Needle	Dose
Retrobulbar eye	2–3 cm 23 g	2% lignocaine + adrenaline +150 units hyaluronidase 3 ml
Tonsillar	Spinal 22 g	1% lignocaine + adrenaline 30 ml total
intravenous Bier	Butterfly or similar 23 g	0.5% lignocaine *plain* 40 ml arm, 60 ml leg
Digital	2–3 cm 23 g	1% lignocaine *plain* 1.5 ml total
Inguinal	2–3 cm 23 g	1% lignocaine + adrenaline 15 ml lat. 15 ml 10 med 40 ml total
Penile	2–3 cm 23 g	1% lignocaine *plain* 15 ml total
Gasserian ganglion	Spinal 22 g	2% lignocaine 2 ml
Ophthalmic nerve	2–3 cm 23 g	2% lignocaine + adrenaline 2 ml
Maxillary nerve	2–3 cm 23 g	2% lignocaine + adrenaline 3 ml
Mandibular nerve	2–3 cm 23–25 g	2% lignocaine + adrenaline 5 ml
Mental nerve	2–3 cm 23–25 g	2% lignocaine + adrenaline 2 ml
Cervical plexus	Spinal 22 g	1% lignocaine + adrenaline 5 ml at each level
Intercostal	2–3 cm 23 g	1% lignocaine + adrenaline 15 ml at each level

Paracervical	Special protected needle	1% lignocaine + adrenaline 15 ml each side
Pudendal	Spinal 22 g	1% lignocaine + adrenaline 15 ml each side
Femoral nerve	Spinal 22 g	1% lignocaine + adrenaline 20 ml
Obturator nerve	Spinal 22 g	1% lignocaine + adrenaline 10 ml
Saphenous nerve	2–3 cm 23 g	1% lignocaine + adrenaline 10 ml
Spinal	Spinal 22 g	0.5% bupivacaine heavy or cinchocaine 1–2.5 ml with positioning
Lumbar epidural	Epidural	1% lignocaine *plain* 15–30 ml; 0.5% bupivacaine *plain* 8–15 ml
Thoracic epidural	Epidural	1% lignocaine *plain* 5–10 ml; 0.5% bupivacaine *plain* 2.5–8 ml
Caudal epidural	3–5 cm 21 g	1% lignocaine *plain* or 0.5% bupivacaine 10–35 ml
Stellate ganglion	Spinal 22 g	1% lignocaine *plain* or 0.5% bupivacaine *plain* 5–10 ml
Lumbar sympathetic	Sympathetic	1% lignocaine *plain* or 0.5% bupivacaine *plain* 5–15 ml
Coeliac ganglion	Sympathetic	1% lignocaine with adrenaline or 0.5% bupivacaine 25–20 ml

The spinal type needles have stilettes and are approximately 7–8 cm 20–22 gauge. The sympathetic type needles have stilettes and are approximately 15–17 cm 18–20 gauge.
We have used lignocaine and bupivacaine in these examples; for doses of other drugs see Section 2.5.1.

2.6 Brachial plexus block

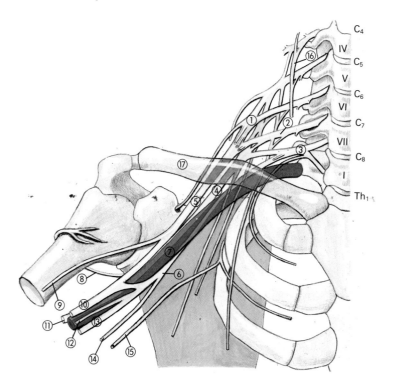

1 Superior trunk.
2 Middle trunk.
3 Inferior trunk.
4 Posterior cord of brachial plexus.
5 Lateral cord of brachial plexus.
6 Medial cord of brachial plexus.
7 Axillary artery.
8 Axillary nerve.
9 Musculocutaneous nerve.
10 Median nerve.
11 Radial nerve.
12 Medial of forearm cutaneous nerve.
13 Ulnar nerve.
14 Medial of arm cutaneous nerve.
15 Intercostobrachial nerve.
16 Phrenic nerve.
17 Clavicle.

2.6.1 Interscalene block

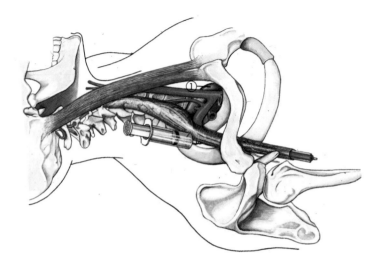

1 Clavicle.
2 Sternomastoid muscle.
3 Anterior scalene muscle.
4 Medial scalene muscle.
5 Interscalene groove, brachial plexus.

6 Perineural sheath.
7 Subclavian artery.
8 Vertebral artery.
9 1. rib.

Indications
Operations on clavicle, shoulder, upper arm, hand and reductions of the shoulder joint.

Special contraindications
Contralateral phrenic paralysis and contralateral recurrent laryngeal nerve paralysis.

Side-effects
Horner's syndrome, phrenic block, recurrent laryngeal nerve block.

Complications
Total spinal anaesthesia, high epidural anaesthesia.

2

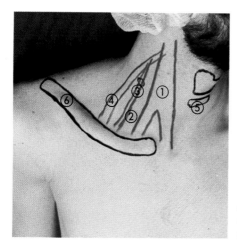

1 Sternocleidomastoid
   muscle.
2 Anterior scalene muscle.
3 Interscalene groove.
4 External jugular vein.
5 Cricoid.
6 Clavicle.

Landmarks
Sternomastoid muscle, interscalene groove, cricoid.

Puncture site
In the interscalene groove, at the level of the cricoid.

Insertion of needle
Medial, caudal (in an angle of 30° to the sagittal plane) and
slightly dorsal, directed to the transverse process of C6.

Dosage
30–40 ml 1% prilocaine (duration 3 h) or 0.375% bupivacaine
(10 h).

2.6.2 Supraclavicular block

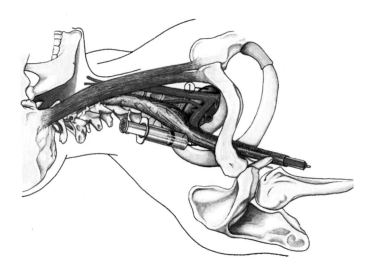

Position of needle, perivascular technique.
1 Dome of pleura.

Indications
Operations of upper arm, lower arm and hand.

Special contraindications
Haemorrhagic diathesis, contralateral phrenic paralysis, contralateral recurrent nerve paralysis, contralateral pneumothorax.

Side-effects
Horner's syndrome, phrenic nerve block, recurrent laryngeal nerve block.

Complications
Pneumothorax, puncture of the subclavian artery.

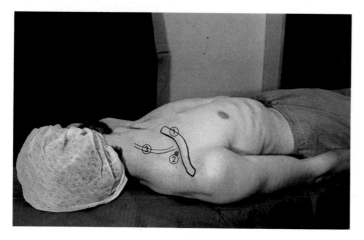

1 Clavicle.
2 Pulsation of subclavian artery.
3 External jugular vein.

Landmarks
Clavicle, subclavian artery.

Puncture site
Immediate dorsolateral from the palpated pulsation of the subclavian artery.

Insertion of needle
Caudal direction and slightly lateral, parallel to the scalene muscles.

Dosage
40 ml 1% prilocaine or 40 ml 0.375% bupivacaine.

2.6.3 Axillary block

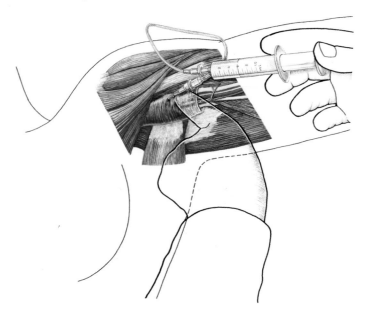

Indications
Operation on lower arm and hand.

Special contraindications
Lymphangitis.

Complications
Puncture of the axillary artery.

2

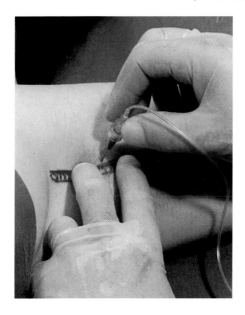

Landmarks
Pulsation of the axillary artery in the axillary groove between the pectoralis major muscle and the latissimus dorsi muscle.

Puncture site
Immediately above the axillary artery, as proximal as possible.

Insertion of needle
Adjacent to axillary artery to enter the perivascular sheath.

Dosage
40 ml 1% prilocaine or 0.375% bupivacaine.

2.7 Peripheral nerve blocks at the elbow

2.7.1 Ulnar nerve

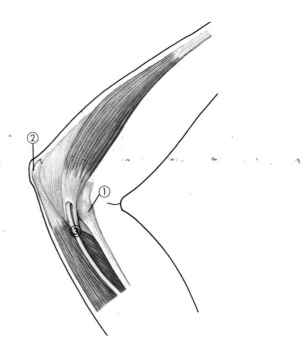

1 Medial epicondyle of humerus.
2 Olecranon.
3 Ulnar nerve.

Indications
Diagnostic, therapeutic and operative interventions in the area of innervation, completion of incomplete brachial plexus block.

Special contraindications
None.

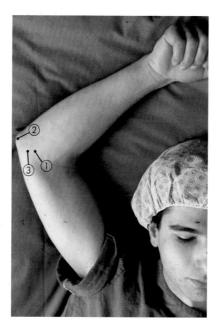

1 Medial epicondyle of humerus.
2 Olecranon.
3 Puncture site.

Landmarks
Medial epicondyle of humerus, olecranon.

Puncture site
1–2 cm proximal from the palpated ulnar nerve in the ulnar groove.

Insertion of needle
Introduce the needle in direction to the longitudinal axis of humerus 1–2 cm deep.

Dosage
2–5 ml 1% prilocaine or 0.5% bupivacaine.

2.7.2 Median nerve

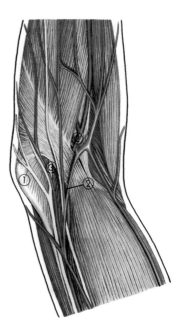

1 Medial epicondyle of humerus.
2 Brachial artery.
3 Median nerve.

Indications
Diagnostic, therapeutic and operative interventions in the area of innervation, completion of incomplete brachial plexus block.

Special contraindications
None.

2

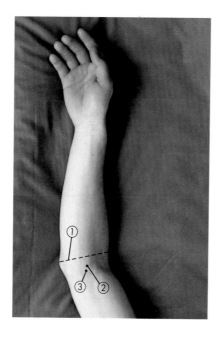

1 Intercondylar line.
2 Brachial artery.
3 Puncture site.

Landmarks
Medial and lateral epicondyles of humerus.

Puncture site
Immediately medial to the brachial artery.

Insertion of needle
Introduce the cannula 5 mm deep.

Dosage
5 ml 1% prilocaine or 0.5% bupivacaine.

2.7.3 Radial nerve

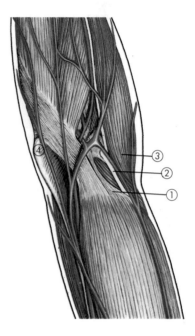

1 Biceps tendon.
2 Radial nerve.
3 Brachioradialis muscle.
4 Medial epicondyle of humerus.

Indications
Diagnostic, therapeutic and operative interventions in the area of innervation, completion of incomplete brachial plexus block.

Special contraindications
None.

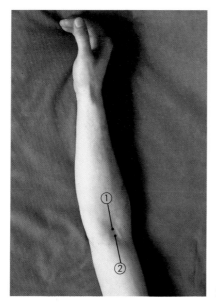

1 Cleft between brachioradialis
  muscle and biceps tendon.
2 Puncture site.

Landmarks
Medial epicondyle of humerus, brachioradialis muscle, biceps
tendon.

Puncture site
In the cleft between the brachioradialis muscle and the biceps
tendon at the level of elbow joint.

Insertion of needle
Push the needle in a proximal and lateral direction to the lateral
margin of lateral epicondyle of humerus. When bone contacted,
infiltrate 2–4 ml local anaesthetic: then advance in a cranial
direction about 1–3 cm in the longitudinal axis of the humerus,
contact the bone again and retract the needle 2–5 mm.

Dosage
10–15 ml 1% prilocaine or 0.5% bupivacaine.

2.8 Peripheral nerve blocks at the wrist

2.8.1 Ulnar nerve

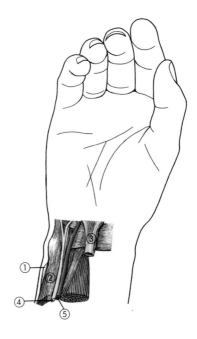

1 Styloid process of ulna.
2 Flexor carpi ulnaris tendon.
3 Palmaris longus tendon.
4 Ulnar nerve.
5 Ulnar artery.

Indications

In combination with median nerve block and radial nerve block, all operations on the hand.

Special contraindications

None.

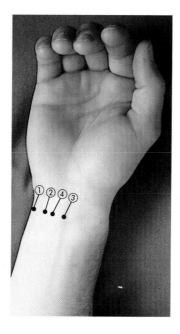

1 Styloid process of ulna.
2 Ulnaris tendon.
3 Palmaris longus tendon.
4 Puncture site.

Landmarks
Flexor carpi ulnaris tendon.

Puncture site
Directly lateral to the flexor carpi ulnaris tendon.

Insertion of needle
Introduce the cannula vertical to the skin 0.5–1 cm deep (if there is a strong resistance to injection, retract 2 mm).

Dosage
2 ml of 1% prilocaine or 0.5% bupivacaine.

2.8.2 Median nerve

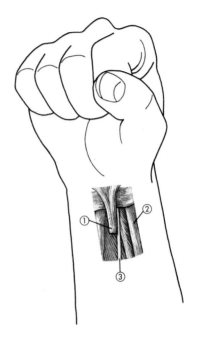

1 Palmaris longus tendon.
2 Flexor carpi radialis tendon.
3 Median nerve.

Indications
In combination with ulnar nerve block and radial nerve block, all operations on the hand.

Special contraindications
None.

2

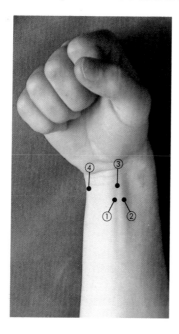

1 Palmaris longus tendon.
2 Flexor carpi radialis tendon.
3 Puncture site.
4 Styloid process of ulna.

Landmarks
Palmaris longus tendon.

Puncture site
Directly lateral to the palmaris longus tendon.

Insertion of needle
Introduce the cannula vertical to the skin 0.5–1 cm deep (if there is a strong resistance to injection, retract 2 mm).

Dosage
2 ml of 1% prilocaine or 0.5% bupivacaine.

2.8.3 Radial nerve

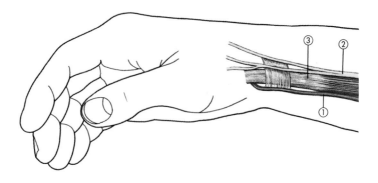

1 Radial artery.
2 Radial nerve.
3 Brachioradialis muscle.

Indications
In combination with ulnar nerve block and median nerve block, all operations on the hand.

Special contraindications
None.

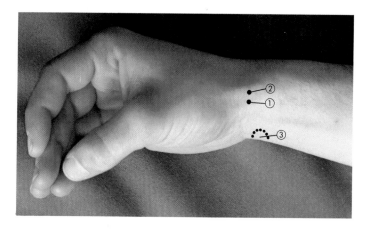

1 Radial artery.
2 Puncture site.
3 Styloid process of ulna.

Landmarks
Pulsation of the radial artery.

Puncture site
About 1 cm lateral to the pulsation of the radial artery.

Insertion of needle
Parallel to the wrist subcutaneously.

Dosage
5 ml 1% prilocaine or 0.25% bupivacaine.

2.9 Sciatic nerve block

2.9.1 Posterior sciatic nerve block

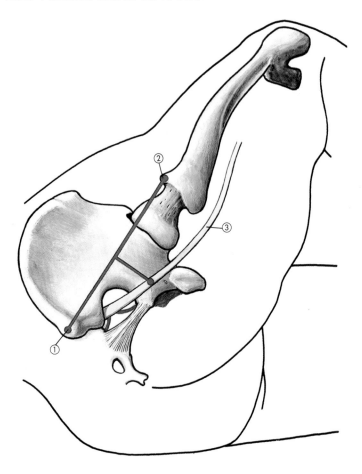

1 Posterior superior iliac spine.
2 Greater trochanter.
3 Sciatic nerve.

2

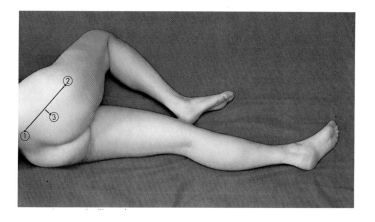

1 Posterior superior iliac spine.
2 Greater trochanter.
3 Puncture site.

Indications
In combination with the 3 in 1 block, all operations on the lower limb.

Special contraindications
None.

Posterior superior iliac spine, greater trochanter.

Puncture site
3 cm below middle of line joining 1 and 2.

Insertion of needle
Introduce the needle vertical to the skin 6–8 cm deep.

Dosage
20–30 ml 1% prilocaine or 0.5% bupivacaine.

2.9.2 Anterior sciatic nerve block

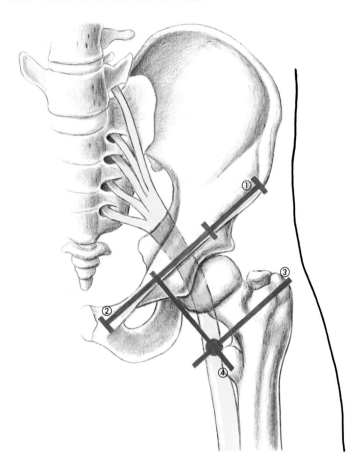

1 Anterior superior iliac spine.
2 Pubic tubercle.
3 Greater trochanter.
4 Sciatic nerve.

2

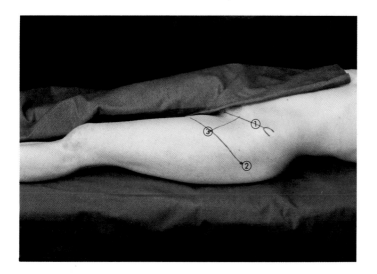

1 Inguinal ligament.
2 Greater trochanter.
3 Puncture site.

Landmarks
Inguinal ligament, greater trochanter.

Puncture site
At the point of intersection of a line from the junction of the middle third and the medial third of the inguinal ligament with a line parallel to the inguinal ligament at the greater trochanter level.

Insertion of needle
Slight lateral direction to contact the femur, retract the needle to the subcutaneous area and correct the direction until the needle glides off the femur, then push forward approx. 5 mm.

Dosage
10–20 ml 1% prilocaine or 0.5% bupivacaine.

2.10 3 in 1 block

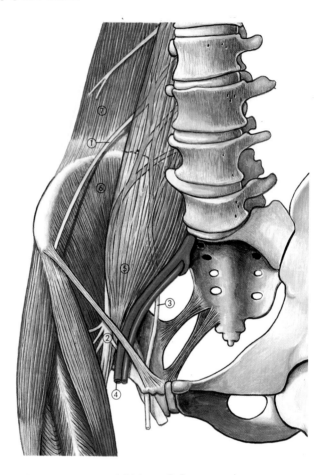

1 Lateral cutaneous nerve of thigh.   5 Psoas muscle.
2 Femoral nerve.   6 Iliac muscle.
3 Obturator nerve.   7 Quadratus lumborum muscle.
4 Femoral artery.

The lumbar plexus is 'sandwiched' (Winnie) between the psoas major muscle and the quadratus lumborum muscle and enveloped by their sheaths.

Local anaesthetic runs up from the injection site and blocks the femoral nerve, the lateral cutaneous nerve of thigh and the obturator nerve.

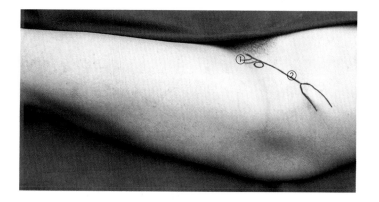

2

1 Femoral artery.
2 Inguinal ligament.

Indications
In combination with sciatic nerve block, all operations on the lower limb.

Special contraindications
None.

Landmarks
Inguinal ligament, femoral artery.

Puncture site
Below the inguinal ligament, 1–1.5 cm lateral from the femoral artery.

Insertion of needle
In slightly cranial direction.

Dosage
25–30 ml 1% prilocaine or 0.5% bupivacaine.

2.11 Peripheral nerve blocks at the knee

2.11.1 Common peroneal nerve

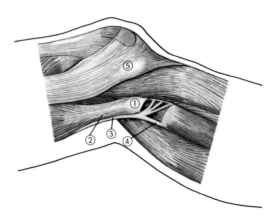

1 Head of fibula.
2 Biceps femoris tendon.
3 Common peroneal nerve.
4 Lateral cutaneous nerve of calf.
5 Lateral condyle of tibia.

Indications
Completion of incomplete peridural anaesthesia or sciatic nerve
block, diagnostic, therapeutic and operative interventions in the
area of innervation, especially fractures of the lateral part of the
ankle and ruptures of the lateral ligament.

Special contraindications
None.

2

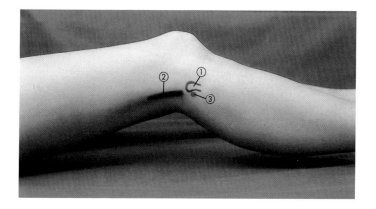

1 Head of fibula.
2 Biceps femoris tendon.
3 Puncture site.

Landmarks
Head of fibula, biceps femoris tendon.

Puncture site
Immediately posterior to fibula, 2 cm below heal.

Insertion of needle
Introduce the needle vertical to the skin approx. 1 cm deep.

Dosage
5 ml 1% prilocaine or 0.5% bupivacaine.

2.11.2 Tibial nerve

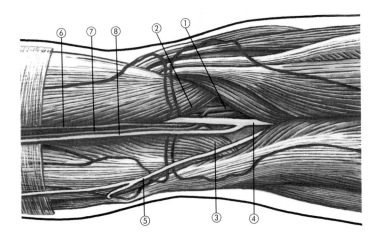

1 Popliteal artery.
2 Medial gastrocnemius muscle.
3 Lateral gastrocnemius muscle.
4 Tibial nerve.

5 Common peroneal nerve.
6 Sural artery.
7 Small saphenous vein.
8 Sural nerve.

Indications

Completion of incomplete peridural anaesthesia or sciatic nerve block; in combination with common peroneal and saphenous nerve block: operations in the area of lower leg and foot.

Special contraindications

None.

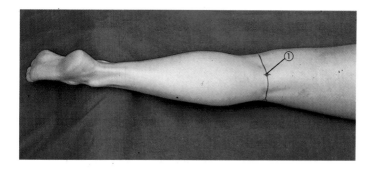

1 Popliteal artery.

Landmarks
Internal and external epicondyles of femur, medial and lateral gastrocnemius muscle.

Puncture site
In the middle of the line connecting the lateral and medial epicondyles of femur.

Insertion of needle
Introduce the needle vertical to the skin 1.5–3 cm deep.

Dosage
5–10 ml 1% prilocaine or 0.5% bupivacaine.

2.11.3 Saphenous nerve

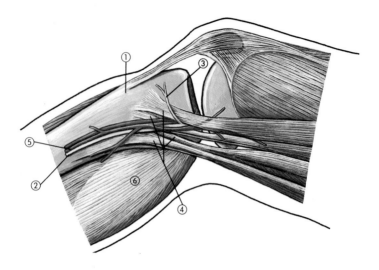

1 Tibial tuberosity.
2 Saphenous nerve.
3 Infrapatellar branch.

4 Pes anserinus.
5 Great saphenous vein.
6 Gastrocnemius muscle.

Indications
Completion of incomplete femoral nerve block, in combination with tibial and fibular nerve block: operations of lower leg and foot.

Special contraindications
None.

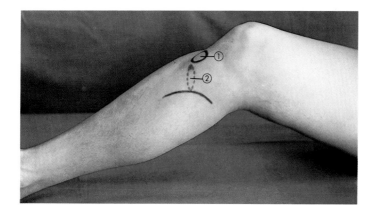

1 Tibial tuberosity.
2 s.c. infiltration.

Landmarks
Medial condyle of tibia, pes anserinus, tibial tuberosity, gastrocnemius muscle.

Puncture site
At the medial part of the tibial tuberosity.

Insertion of needle
s.c. infiltration from the medial part of the tibial tuberosity to the gastrocnemius muscle.

Dosage
5–10 ml 1% prilocaine or 0.5% bupivacaine.

2.12 Foot block

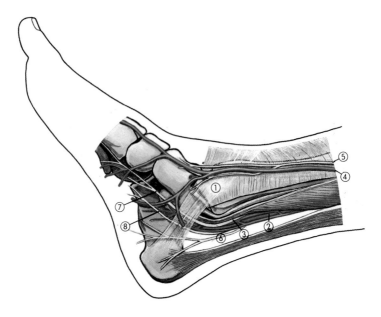

1 Medial malleolus.
2 Tibial artery.
3 Tibial nerve.
4 Great saphenous vein.

5 Saphenous nerve.
6 Medial calcanean branch.
7 Medial plantar nerve.
8 Lateral plantar nerve.

Indications
All operations of foot and toes.

Special contraindications
None.

2

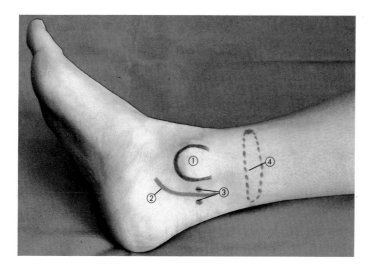

1 Medial malleolus.
2 Tibial artery.
3 Puncture sites (tibial nerve block).
4 s.c. infiltration (saphenous nerve block).

Landmarks
Medial malleolus, tibial artery.

Puncture sites
On both sides of the tibial artery.

Insertion of needle
Introduce the needle vertical to the skin 0.5–2 cm deep.

Dosage
2–3 ml of 1% prilocaine or 0.5% bupivacaine.

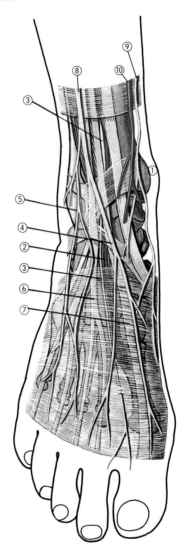

1 Medial malleolus.
2 Dorsalis pedis artery.
3 Deep peroneal nerve.
4 Medial branch of superficial peroneal nerve.
5 Lateral branch of superficial peroneal nerve.
6 Extensor digitorum longus tendon.
7 Extensor hallucis longus tendon.
8 Superficial peroneal nerve.
9 Saphenous nerve.
10 Great saphenous vein.

2

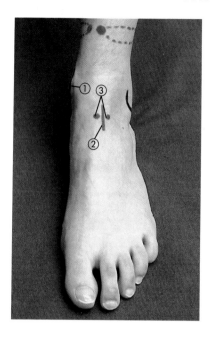

1 Medial malleolus.
2 Dorsalis pedis artery.
3 Puncture sites (deep peroneal
  nerve block).

Landmarks
Dorsalis pedis artery.

Puncture sites
On both sides of dorsalis pedis artery.

Insertion of needle
Introduce the needle vertical to the skin directly beside the artery,
up to slightly below it. Repeat on other side of artery.

Dosage
2–3 ml of 1% prilocaine or 0.5% bupivacaine for each injection.

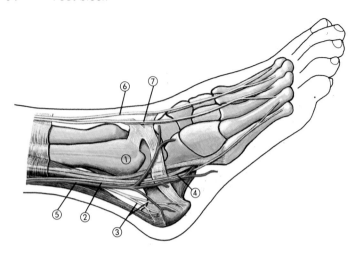

1 Lateral malleolus.
2 Sural nerve.
3 Lateral calcanael branch.
4 Lateral dorsal cutaneous nerve.
5 Small saphenous vein.
6 Medial branch of superior peroneal nerve.
7 Lateral branch of superior peroneal nerve.

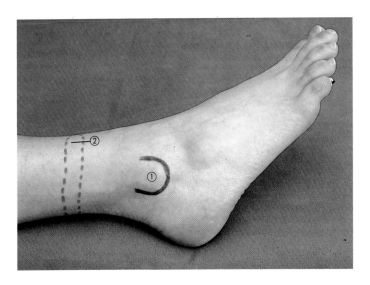

1 Lateral malleolus.
2 s.c. infiltration.

Landmarks
Lateral malleolus, tibial edge, achilles tendon.

Insertion of needle
s.c. infiltration from the tibial edge to the achilles tendon about one hand's breadth above the lateral malleolus.
s.c. infiltration from the tibial edge to the achilles tendon about one hand's breadth above the medial malleolus.

Dosage
10–20 ml of 1% prilocaine or 0.25%–0.5% bupivacaine.

Section 3
Burns

3

3.1 Lund and Bowder chart for accurate assessment of percentages of body surface area

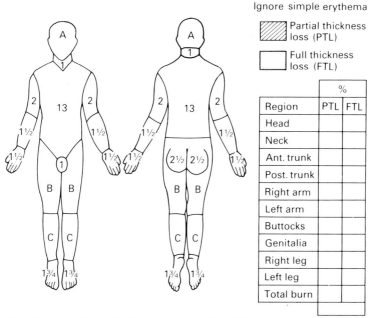

Ignore simple erythema

Partial thickness loss (PTL)

Full thickness loss (FTL)

3

Region	PTL	FTL
Head		
Neck		
Ant. trunk		
Post. trunk		
Right arm		
Left arm		
Buttocks		
Genitalia		
Right leg		
Left leg		
Total burn		

Relative percentage of body surface area affected by growth

Area	Age 0	1	5	10	15	Adult
A = ½ of head	9½	8½	6½	5½	4½	3½
B = ½ of one thigh	2¾	3¼	4	4½	4½	4¾
C = ½ of one leg	2½	2½	2¾	3	3¼	3½

3.2 Guide to immediate treatment of burns

1 Assess burn.
2 If burn is less than 10% BSA use oral solution of 1 litre of normal saline + 1 litre of tap water + 100 ml 1.26% $NaHCO_3$ + orange juice flavouring. Give 10% wt in litres divided over 24–36 hours.
3 If burn is more than 10% BSA use i.v. fluids, 0.5 ml/kg % burn, given in each period shown below, as HPPF

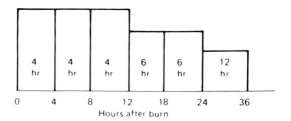

4 Calculate plasma deficit every 4 hours and adjust fluid input accordingly.

$$\text{Plasma deficit} = \text{blood volume} - \left(\text{blood volume} \times \frac{\text{normal HCT}}{\text{measured HCT}}\right).$$

5 If burn is over 10% BSA give 1% blood volume × % burn as blood within the second 24 hour period.

6 Give 1.5 ml/kg/h of water i.v. or orally for the metabolic water needs.

7 Catheterize patient. Urine should be 0.5–1 ml/kg/h with an osmolarity of more than 800 mosmol/l. Mannitol 1 g/kg if oliguria or haemaglobinuria present.

8 Adequate analgesia is always needed, often in large doses, to avoid systematic effects of severe pain. Morphine, papaveretum or pethidine are indicated. Satisfactory pain relief may be gained by continuous infusion of these drugs.

9 Nasogastric tube inserted with ranitidine given. Give high calorie and protein diet when possible. Monitor blood sugar. Burned patients may have inhaled chemical irritants, steam, or super-heated air. Frequent monitoring of respiration, clinical and biochemical status is needed to anticipate deterioration. Nurse in clean area and treat infections.

Section 4
Clinical Biochemistry and Haematology

4

4.1 Normal blood values

Normal values tend to vary from laboratory to laboratory,
depending on reagents and techniques used. We have taken these
figures from many sources; if in doubt contact your own
laboratory.

4.1.1 Biochemistry normals

4

Name	Value in SI units	Value in old units
Acetone	51.6–344 μmol	0.3–2 mg%
Aldolase	0.5–3.1 iu/l	0.9–2.5 iu/l
Amino acid nitrogen	3–6 mmol/l	4–8 mg%
Ammonia	10–40 μmol/l	20–50 μg/%
Amylase	70–30 iu/l	80–180 Somogyi u%
Arsenic	0.67–1.3 μmol	5–10 μg/%
Alanine amino transferase	23 iu/l	
Base excess	±2 mmol/l	±2 mEq/l
Bicarbonate		
actual	24–32 mmol/l	24–32 mEq/l
standard	21–25 mmol/l	21–25 mEq/l
Bilirubin		
total	3–18 μmol/l	0.3–1.1 mg%
conjugated	<7 μmol/l	<0.4 mg%
Bromide	0.7–1.33 μmol/l	0.7–1.3 μg%
Bromsulphthalein (BSP)		<5% after 45 min, giving 5 mg/kg i.v.
Buffer base	48 mmol/l (pH 7.4: P_{CO_2} 40)	48 mEq/l
Cadmium	0.027–0.045 μmol/l	0.3–0.5 μg%
Caeruloplasmin	300–600 mg/l	30–60 mg%
Calcium		
total	2.25–2.6 mmol/l	8.5–10.5 mg% (4.5–5.7 mEq)
ionized	1–1.25 mmol/l	4.5 mg%
Carbon dioxide		
P_vCO_2	5.3–6.9 kPa	40–52 mmHg
P_aCO_2	4.5–6.1 kPa	34–46 mmHg
content	48–52 ml%	48–52 ml%
Carotenoids	1.8–5.5 μmol/l	100–300 μg/l
Catecholamines	<54.6 nmol/l	1 μg%
Chloride	95–105 mmol/l	95–105 mEq/l
Cholesterol	3.6–7.8 mmol/l	140–300 mg/l
Cholesterol (HDL)	>1 mmol/l	
Cholesterol (LDL)	<4.5 mmol/l	

Name	Value in SI units	Value in old units
Cholestinerase		
acetyl	9–25 µmol/ml/min	
plasma		40–100 units%
Chromium		2–6 µg%
Copper	13–24 nmol/l	80–150 µg%
Cobalt	50.7 nmol/l	0.3 µg%
Cortisol		
0900 h	250–650 nmol/l	9–23 µg%
2400 h	< 200 nmol/l	< 7.2 µg%
	828 nmol/l	
Creatine	15.2–60.8 µmol/l	0.2–0.8 mg%
Creatinephosphokinase	< 60 iu/l ♂	100 iu/l
	< 60 iu/l ♀	60 iu/l
Creatinine	45–120 µmol/l	0.5–1.4 mg%
Fibrinogen	2.0–5 g/l	200–500 mg%
Folate	3–20 µg/l	3–20 ng/ml
Fluoride	7.4–10 µmol/l	0.014–0.019 mg%
Glucose		
fasting	3–4.6 mmol/l	55–85 mg%
postprandial	< 10 mmol/l	< 180 mg%
γ-glutamyl transferase	10–45 iu/l	7–28 iu/l
Glycogen storage	Blood sugar 2.5 mmol/l over fasting level, 45 min after subcut. inject. of epinephrine 0.01 mg/kg	
Gold		0.1–40 µg%
2-hydroxybutyrate		
dehydrogenase (HBD)	500–1 300 iu/l	50–130 iu%
Iodine 131 uptake		20–50% of administered dose in 24 h
Iron	6–25 µmol/l	80–160 µg%
Iron binding capacity	45–72 µmol/l	250–400 µg%
Isocitric dehydrogenase		
(ICD)	20–140 iu/l	2–4 iu
Ketones (as acetone)	80–140 µmol/l	0.8–1.4 mg%
Lactate	0.6–2.4 mmol/l	3.6–15 mg%
Lactic dehydrogenase		
(LDH)	30–90 iu/l	100–300 iu
Lead	< 1.2 µmol/l	10–40 µg%
Lipase		0–15 µ/ml
Lipids		
total	4–10 g/l	400–1000 mg%
S particles	0–5.5 g/l	0.550 mg%
M particles	0–2.4 g/l	0–240 mg%
L particles	0–0.28 g/l	0–28 mg%
Magnesium	0.7–1.1 mmol/l	1.8–2.4 mg% 1.4–2.8 mEq/l
Manganese	40 nmol/l	2.2 µg/l

Name	Value in SI units	Value in old units
Methaemoglobin	0.1–5 g/l	0.01–0.5 g%
Mercury	0–0.25 µmol/l	0–5 µg%
Nicotinic acid	0.13–0.41 µmol/l	0.0016–0.005 mg%
Nitrogen (non-protein)	12.8–21.4 mmol/l	18–30 mg%
Nickel	0–1 µmol/l	6.3 µg%
Noradrenaline	2.95 nmol/l	0.05 µg%
5-Nucleotidase	1.5–17 iu/l	1.5–17 iu/l
Osmolality	280–300 mosmol/kg	280–300 mosmol/kg
pH venous	38–48 nmol/l	7.32–7.42
pH ⎫	36–44 nmol/l (H$^+$ ion)	7.36–7.45
P_{CO_2} ⎬ arterial	4.5–6.1 kPa	34–46
P_{O_2} ⎭	12–15 kPa	90–110 mmHg
Phenylalanine	0.06–0.2 mmol/l	1–3 mg%
Phosphate (inorganic)	0.64–1.4 mmol/l	2–4.5 mg%
	1–1.8 mmol/l	
	in children	
Phosphatase		
acid	1–7 iu/l (37°C)	1–5 KA unit
alkaline	20–90 iu/l (37°C)	3–13 KA unit
	< 150 in children	
Phospholipids	1.6–3.2 mmol/l	5–10 mg%
Potassium	3.8–5 mmol/l	15–20 mg% 3.8–5.0 mEq/l
Protein		
total	62–80 g/l	6.2–8 g%
albumin	36–47 g/l	3.6–4.7 g%
globulin	24–37 g/l	2.4–3.7 g%
IgA ⎫	1.5–3.5 g/l	150–350 mg%
IgG ⎬ adult	7–18 g/l	700–1800 mg%
IgM ⎪	0.5–2.1 g/l	50–205 mg% ∫
IgD ⎭		0.3–40 mg%
Pyruvate	45–80 µmol/l	0.4–0.7 mg%
Sodium	135–148 mmol/l	306–329 mg% 135–148 mEq/l
Serotonin		0.1–0.35 µg/ml
Sulphate	0.312–0.56 mmol/l	1–18 mg%
Thymol turbidity	0–3 units/ml	0–3 units/ml
Thyroxine-iodine T$_4$	69–150 nmol	5–12 µg%
Transaminase		
SGOT	4–18 iu/l	0–40 units/ml
SGPT	< 23 iu/l	0–12 units/ml
Triglycerides	0.34–1.7 mmol/l	30–150 mg%
Transferrin	1.2–2 g/l	120–200 mg%
TSH	0.6–6.5 mu/l	
Tyrosine	27.6–110 µmol/l	0.5–2 mg%
T$_3$ absolute	0.8–2.5 nmol/l	
FT$_4$	8–24 pmol/l	
FT$_3$	3–9 pmol/l	

Name	Value in SI units	Value in old units
T_3 uptake	95–115%	95–115%
T_4 free	8.24 pmol/l	
Urea	2.5–6.5 mmol/l	15–40 mg%
Urea nitrogen	1.66–3.3 mmol/l	10–20 mg%
Urate	0.1–0.4 mmol/l	2–7 mg%
Vitamin		
A	0.7–1.7 µmol/l	20–50 µg%
B_1	33.2 nmol/l	1 µg%
B_2	0.008–0.0346 µmol/l	0.3–1.3 µg%
B_6	0.18–0.48 µmol/l	3–8 µg%
B_{12}	150–1000 ng/l	
C	28.0–84 µmol/l	0.5–1.5 mg%
D	1.79–7.69 mmol/l	70–300 mg%
E	13.18–45.9	560–1950 µg%
Volume		
blood		49–75 ml/kg body wt ♂;
		56–75 ml/kg body wt ♀
		2500–400 ml/m²
plasma		31–55 ml/kg body wt ♂;
		36–50 ml/kg body wt ♀
		1400–2500 ml/m²
red cell		18–33 ml/kg body wt ♂;
		20–27 ml/kg body wt ♀
Zinc	0.5–1 mmol/l	1–2 mEq/l
Zinc turbidity		2–6 units

4.1.2 Routine haematology

All the samples below are collected in an EDTA (sequestrene) bottle.

Haemoglobin (Hb)	men	13.5–18 g/dl
	women	11.5–16.5 g/dl
Red blood cell count (RBC)	men	$4.5–6 \times 10^{12}/l$
	women	$3.5–5 \times 10^{12}/l$
White blood cell count (WBC)		$4–11 \times 10^9/l$
neutrophils	40–75%	$2.5–7.5 \times 10^9/l$
lymphocytes	20–45%	$1.5–3.5 \times 10^9/l$
monocytes	2–10%	$0.2–0.8 \times 10^9/l$
eosinophils	1–6%	$0.04–0.44 \times 10^9/l$
basophils	0–1%	$0–0.1 \times 10^9/l$
Platelet count		$150–400 \times 10^9/l$
Reticulocyte count	0–2%	of RBCs
Sedimentation rate (ESR)	men	3–5 mm in first hour
	women	4–7 mm in first hour
Packed cell volume (PCV)	men	0.40–0.55
Haematocrit (HCT)	women	0.36–0.47
Mean corpuscular volume (MCV)		76–96 fl
Mean corpuscular haemoglobin concentration (MCHC)		31–35 g/dl
Mean corpuscular haemoglobin (MCH)		27–32 pg

Haptoglobin binding capacity is usually above 1 g of haemoglobin per litre of plasma. The lower and upper limits of 'normal' vary widely depending on the clinical state.

Miscellaneous tests
Serum
vitamin B12	150–1000 ng/l
folic acid	3–20 µg/l

Sequestrene (EDTA)
red cell folate	160–640 µg/l

Plasma (heparin tube)
iron	14–30 µmol/l
total iron binding capacity (TIBC)	45–69 µmol/l

4.2 Management of the bleeding patient

When patients bleed unexpectedly, it is always wise to consult a haematologist. Blood tests are only of real value when the following questions have been answered:

1 Why is the patient bleeding now?
2 Has abnormal bleeding occurred before?
3 What drugs are being used or have been taken recently?
4 Is there a family history of.abnormal bleeding?
5 Are there abnormal physical signs?
  a purpura?
  b palpable nodes, liver or spleen?
  c evidence of previous haemorrhage into joints or muscles?

4.2.1 Coagulation tests

Platelet count: 150 400 × 10^9/l.

Bleeding time: 2 9 minutes
The result of this test varies depending on the site chosen and the method used. A commercial template method is available which helps to standardize the result.

Coagulation or clotting time: 3 11 minutes
The result of this obsolete test varies depending on the method used.

Samples for the following tests are collected in citrate tubes. The figures quoted are only guides to the normal ranges which vary between laboratories.

Prothrombin time (PT): 14 18 seconds
This test measures deficiency of factors I, II, V, VII, X (extrinsic system).

Prothrombin ratio (PTR):

$$1 1.3 = \frac{PT}{control}$$

Prothrombin ratios are now widely standardized by use of comparative thromboplastins, and the result is expressed as the International Normalized Ratio (INR). The therapeutic range for oral anticoagulants is approx. 2–4.5. The prothrombin ratio is also useful in the diagnosis of hepatic dysfunction.

Thrombotest: Therapeutic range 5–15%
This is a commercial variant of the prothrombin ratio and is used to monitor oral anticoagulants in some centres.

4

Partial thromboplastin time (PTT): 35–45 seconds
This test measures deficiencies of factors I, II, V, X, VIII, IX, XI, XII (intrinsic system). The most common variant of this test is the kaolin cephalin clotting time test (KCCT) which uses kaolin as an activator and cephalin as a platelet phospholipid substitute. The normal range given above is wide and varies between laboratories. The test is useful for analysis of hereditary clotting defects, intravascular coagulation and monitoring heparin therapy.

Thrombin clotting time (TCT, TT)
Calcium thrombin clotting time: 10–20 seconds. Sensitive to hypofibrinogenaemia, heparin and fibrinogen degradation products. The test is used for diagnosis of intravascular coagulation and to monitor heparin therapy.
Reptilase time: 17–20 seconds. Sensitive to hypofibrinogenaemia and fibrinogen degradation products but normal in the presence of heparin. The test is useful in the diagnosis of intravascular coagulation especially in the presence of heparin.
Fibrinogen: 2–4 g/l. This is useful in the diagnosis of intravascular coagulation.
Fibrinogen degradation products (FDP): < 10 mg/l. This test is useful in the diagnosis of intravascular coagulation. Note: the blood is collected in a tube containing thrombin to which EACA has been added, although one slightly different method now uses citrated plasma.
Euglobulin lysis time: > 2 hours. This measures fibrinolytic activator in the blood and is used in the assessment of fibrinolytic status.

4.2.2 Haemostasis tests

The table of screening tests opposite gives a rough guide to diagnosis and management of the bleeding patient.

Please note:

1 It is always worthwhile to discuss the results of tests with a haematologist. The problems of further investigation and treatment are often complex and normal routine test results do not rule out a haemostatic defect in all cases.

2 When serious haemorrhage has taken place, it may be difficult to distinguish a primary haemostatic defect from the secondary effect of bleeding and blood transfusion.

3 Where there is an established or suspected defect of haemostasis, intramuscular injection should be avoided.

4 Blood samples from patients and from some therapeutic blood products may carry a risk of viral infection to the clinical and laboratory staff. Special care should be taken in the management of high risk patients.

4

Abnormality	Possible diagnosis	Possible management
Platelets reduced; clotting tests normal	Bone marrow failure, e.g. aplasia, malignancy, vitamin deficiency Consumption of platelets, e.g. ITP, hypersplenism	Specific therapy, e.g. folic acid, withdrawal of causative drugs Platelet infusions, corticosteroids, immunosuppression
PTR only abnormal	Exclude presence of oral anticoagulants and liver disease. Factor VII deficiency rare	If presence of oral anticoagulants is confirmed then consider, FFP, vitamin K and/or factor concentrates
PTT only abnormal	Probable inherited defect of intrinsic pathway, e.g. haemophilia or von Willebrand's disease. In the latter, platelet function is defective, with long bleeding time	After confirming with specific factor assays, give specific factor concentrates DDAVP or other treatment as advised by a haematologist
PTR, PTT abnormal, TCT and platelets normal	Typical of oral anticoagulants, liver disease, vitamin K deficiency. Exclude DIC, and inherited defects of II, V, X, which are rare	Vitamin K, FFP, and/or factor concentrates

Abnormality	Possible diagnosis	Possible management
PTR, PTT abnormal, TCT normal, platelets reduced	Massive blood transfusion. Exclude DIC and liver disease	FFP and platelet concentrates especially when platelets $<50 \times 10^9/l$ or PTR > 1.8
PTR, PTT, TCT abnormal: reptilase and platelets normal	Typical of heparin therapy (or see below)	Exclude haemostatic failure due to heparin. Consider withdrawing heparin or using protamine
All clotting tests abnormal. Platelets normal or reduced: red cells fragmented on film	Typical of severe liver disease or DIC	Avoid factor concentrates if possible* In liver disease use vitamin K and FFP. In DIC use FFP, platelet concentrates ±heparin, after trying to treat underlying condition†

*Factor concentrates may be dangerous because of the possibility of exacerbating DIC.
†Antifibrinolytic agents should be confined to those patients who show abnormal proteolytic activity in the absence of DIC. They are generally contraindicated in bleeding from the upper renal tract.

4.3 Normal urinary values

Name	Values in SI units (per 24 h)	Values in old units (per 24 h)
Adrenaline	0.05–0.85 µmol	10–150 µg
Ammonium	17.7–59 mmol	0.03–1 g
Amylase	170–2000 µl	
Ascorbic acid	85–284 µmol	15–50 mg
Amino acid nitrogen	4–20 mmol	50–300 mg
5-Aminolaevulate	0.8–46 µmol	0.1–6 mg
Aldosterone	<43 nmol	<15 µg
Calcium	2.5–7.5 mmol	100–300 mg
Chloride	100–300 mmol	100–300 mEq
Cortisol	0.36–0.99 µmol ($\male$)	130–360 µg
	0.19–0.77 µmol ($\female$)	
	0.05–0.85 µmol	20–150 µg
Creatine	0–760 µmol (adult)	0–100 mg
	68 µmol/kg (neonate)	
Creatinine	8.85–17.7 mmol	1–2 g
Creatinine clearance		120 ml/min
Copper	0.2–0.8 µmol	10–50 µg
Coproporphyrin	150–300 nmol	100–200 µg
Cysteine	42–420 µmol	
Folic acid		3.5–23.5 µg
Formiminoglutamate	0–170 µmol	0–30 mg
Galactose tolerance test		<3 g in urine 5 h post-ingestion of 40 g galactose
Glomerular filtration rate		105–140 ml/min
Glucose	0–11 mmol/l	0–0.2 g%
Hydroxyproline	0.08–0.25 mmol	10–30 mg/g creatinine
5-Hydroxyindole acetic acid (5HIAA)	15–75 µmol	3–14 mg
4-Hydroxy-3-methoxy mandelate (HMMA)	10–35 µmol	2–7 mg
Iodine 131 excretion		30–70% of adminis-tered dose in 24 h
Iron	1–18 µmol	0.06–1 mg
17 Ketosteroids	34.7–104 µmol	10–30 mg
Lead	0.14–0.40 µmol	30–80 µg
Magnesium	3.3–5 mmol	80–120 mg
Mercury	0–498 nmol	0–100 µg

Name	Values in SI units (per 24 h)	Values in old units (per 24 h)
Nitrogen non-protein	0.7–1.43 mmol	10–20 g
Noradrenaline	29.6–592 nmol	5–100 µg
Normetadrenaline	0–5.5 nmol	0–1 mg
Oestriol (after 30 week pregnancy)	30–140 µmol	8–40 mg
Oestrogens	14–86.7 µmol	4–25 µg ♂
	14–347 µmol	4–100 µg non-pregnant ♀
Osmolality	300–1000 mosmol/kg	300–1000 mosmol/kg
Oxalate	0.2–0.4 mmol	20–40 mg
17 Oxogenic steroids	30–79 µmol	10–20 mg
17 Oxosteroids	30–85 µmol	8–25 mg
Phosphate	15–50 mmol	0.5–1.5 g
Potassium	30–100 mmol	30–100 mEq
Protein (albumin)		0–0.1 g
Pregnandiol	0–3.1 µmol	0–10 mg
pH	30 000–10 nmol	<5.3
Phosphatase		
acid		164 KA units (♂)
		217 KA units (♀)
alkaline		<6000 KA units (♂)
		<7500 KA units (♀)
Porphobilinogen	1–10 µmol	0.2–2 mg
Pregnantriol	0.3–9 µmol	0.1–3 mg
Renal plasma flow		500–800 ml/min
Sodium	50–200 mmol	50–200 mEq
Specific gravity		1003–1030
Sulphur (as SO_3)	21.7–108.5 mmol	0.7–3.5 g
Urea	249–581 mmol	15–35 g
Urea clearance		60–95 ml/min
Urate	1.2–4.4 mmol	0.2–0.74 g
Urobilinogen	0–6.7 µmol	0–4 mg
Uroporphyrin I and III	0–30 nmol	0–25 µg
Volume	1–1.8 l	1–1.8 l
VMA		1.6 µg/mg of creatinine

4.4 Normal CSF values

CSF is normally clear and colourless with the following characteristics.

	Values in SI units	Values in old units	Remarks
Pressure	0.69–1.47	70–150 mmH$_2$O	
Volume	120–140	120–140 ml	
pH	50–54 mmol/l	7.30–7.35	(H$^+$ ion)
Lymphocytes	0–5 × 10^6/l	0–5 mm^3	
Specific gravity	1007	1007	
Osmolality	306 mosmol/kg	306 mosmol/kg	
Calcium	1–1.5 mmol/l	2–3 mEq/l	
Chloride	120–130 mmol/l	120–130 mEq/l	
Glucose	2.2–4.5 mmol/l	40–80 mg%	1.1 mmol/l less than blood sugar
Magnesium	0.36–3.2 mmol/l	0.45–4 mEq/l	
Phosphate	0.13–0.23 mmol/l	0.4–0.7 mEq/l	
Potassium	3–4 mmol/l	3–4 mEq/l	
Protein	150–400 mg/l	15–40 mg%	
globulin	0–20 mg/l	0–2 mg%	
Sodium	140 mmol/l	140 mEq/l	
Urea	1.33–6.64 mmol/l	8–40 mg%	
IgG	5.45 mg/l (adult) 0.8–6.4 mg/l (child)		

4.5 Normal stool values

	Values in SI units (per 24 h)	Values in old units (per 24 h)
Bulk	100–200 g	100–200 g
Dry weight	23–32 g	23–32 g
Water content	65%	65%
Fat total	<25 mmol (adult) <15 mmol (child)	<5 g
Nitrogen	70–140 mmol	1–2 g
Urobilinogen	50–500 μmol	30–300 mg

Section 5
Critical Care and Resuscitation

5

5.1 Guidelines for assessment and resuscitation of patients with multiple injuries

5.1.1 Initial assessment

Airway
1 Clear mouth of obstructing material.
2 Remember possible cervical spine injury.
3 Relieve anatomical obstruction by positioning of airway.
4 Intubate if necessary with suction available.

5

Breathing
1 Provide adequate oxygenation.
2 If no spontaneous breathing: ventilate, preferably after intubation, if not by mask or mouth to mouth ventilation.
3 Check:
   chest movement in and out
   possible pneumothorax
   possible haemothorax
   possible flail segment

Circulation
1 Pulse present?
   femoral
   radial
   carotid
2 Measure blood pressure:
   if no circulation, cardiac massage
   if circulation inadequate, stop obvious haemorrhage

Establish intravenous infusion
1 Restore blood volume with:
   blood plasma, protein fraction
   plasma expander: Hespan, Haemaccel or Gelofusin
2 If circulation still inadequate:
   consider concealed haemorrhage
   consider inotropic support if blood volume restored
If possible, establish large bore central venous pressure line and arterial line.

Take blood samples

1 Measure:
   haemoglobin, haematocrit
   urea, electrolytes
   blood sugar
   liver function tests
   arterial blood gases
2 Cross match 6 units of whole blood.

Establish ECG monitor
(if not already attached)

5.1.2 Secondary assessment

1 Look for:
   pneumothorax
   haemothorax
   flail chest
   cardiac tamponade
   concealed haemorrhage in mediastinum, abdomen, limbs and
   pelvis
2 Baseline neurological examination:
   pupils
   Glasgow coma score
3 Reassess:
   breathing
   circulation
   blood loss
4 X-ray:
   chest
   skull
   cervical spine
   pelvis
   limbs
5 Unless contraindicated or unnecessary pass:
   nasogastric tube
   urethral catheter

5.1.3 Third check

Reassessment
Airway
Breathing
Circulation
Blood loss
Transfusion

Full neurological examination

Thorax
1 Consider rupture of:
aorta
oesophagus
tracheo-bronchi
diaphragm
2 Consider contusion of:
heart
lung

Abdomen
1 Consider rupture of:
spleen
liver
gut
aorta
bladder
urethra
2 Fractured pelvis.

5

5.2 Cardiac arrest procedure

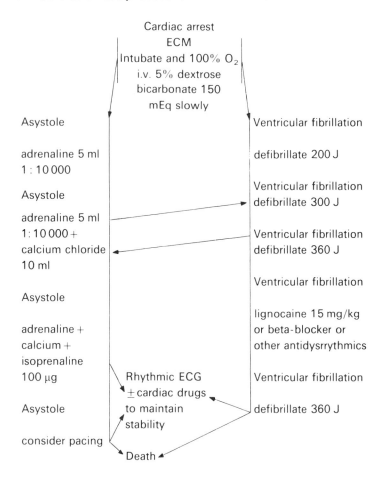

Pulmonary oedema is treated with frusemide 1 mg/kg.
Cerebral oedema is treated with mannitol 15–20 g
Renal shutdown is treated with mannitol or frusemide as above
See p. 104 for treatment of arrythmias

5.3 Assessment of coma severity

5.3.1 Glasgow coma scale

From Jennett, B. & Bond, M. (1975) Assessment of outcome after severe brain injury. *Lancet*, **ii**, 480.

Eyes open		Spontaneously	4
		To verbal command	3
		To pain	2
		No response	1
Best motor response	To verbal command	Obeys	6
	To painful stimulus	Localizes	5
		Flexion—withdrawal	4
		Flexion—abnormal (decorticate rigidity)	3
		Extension (decerebrate rigidity)	2
		No response	1
Best verbal response		Orientated, converses	5
		Disorientated, converses	4
		Inappropriate words	3
		Incomprehensible sounds	2
		No response	1

5.4 APACHE II: Acute physiology and chronic health evaluation

APACHE II (Knaus, W. A., Draper, E. A., Wagner, D. P. & Zimmerman, J. A. (1985). APACHE II: a severity of disease classification system. *Critical Care Medicine*, **13**, 818–29.) is the most widely accepted acute physiology scoring system in use in the UK and the USA. It is a scoring system based on twelve physiological variables, age and previous health record.

Although originally described to score the worst value for each parameter in the first 24 hours of admission, it can also be used for a scoring evaluation on admission before treatment and evaluation of a patient's progress during admission, and any comparison between patients must state the circumstances of the measurement.

An increasing score is closely related to a deteriorating prognosis and can be used to measure progress, prognosis and use of hospital resources, and to compare the performance of different intensive therapy units.

5.4.1 The APACHE II severity of disease classification system

Physiological variable	Points				Normal				
	High abnormal range					Low abnormal range			
	+4	+3	+2	+1	0	+1	+2	+3	+4
Temperature: rectal °C	>41	39–40.9		38.5–38.9	36–38.4	34–35.9	32–33.9	30–31.9	<29.9
Mean arterial pressure (mmHg) $\frac{(2 \times \text{diastolic} + \text{systolic})}{3}$	>160	130–159	110–129		70–109		50–69		<49
Heart rate (ventricular response)	>180	140–179	110–139		70–109		55–69	40–54	<39
Respiratory rate (non-ventilated or ventilated)	>50	35–49		25–34	12–24	10–11	8–9		<5
Oxygenation If $FiO_2 > 0.5$ record (A–a) DO_2 mmHg = $FiO_2 \times 713 - PaCO_2 - PaO_2$	≥500	350–499	200–349		<200				
OR kPa = $FiO_2 \times 94.8 - PaCO_2 - PaO_2$	≥66.8	46.7–66.5	26.7–46.5		<26.7				
If $FiO_2 < 0.5$ record PaO_2					>70mmHg	61–7		55–60	<55
					>9.3 kPa	8.1–9.3		7.3–8.0	<7.3
Arterial pH	>7.7	7.6–7.69		7.5–7.59	7.33–7.49	7.25–7.32		7.15–7.24	<7.15
OR									

Serum HCO_3 (venous mmol/l)*	>52	41–51.9		32–40.9	22–31.9		18–21.9	15–17.9	<15
Serum sodium (mmol/l)	>180	160–179	155–159	150–154	130–149		120–129	111–119	<110
Serum potassium (mmol/l)	>7	6–6.9		5.5–5.9	3.5–5.4	3–3.4	2.5–2.9		<2.5
Serum creatinine (double points for renal failure)									
mg/100 ml	>3.5	2–3.4	1.5–1.9				<0.6		
µmol/l	>309	177–308	133–176		53–132		<53		
Haematocrit (%)	>60		50–59.9	46–49.9	30–45.9		20–29.9		<20
White blood count (total/mm³ in 1000 s)	>40		20–39.9	15–19.9	3–14.9		1–2.9		<1
Glasgow coma score (GCS) (score = 15-GCS)									

* Use only if no ABG—assume normal oxygen.

A Total acute physiology score (APS) = sum of the 12 variables above.

B Age points: assign points to age as follows:

Age (yr)	Points
⩽44	0
45–54	2
55–64	3
65–74	5
⩾75	6

5

(*Footnotes for table continued*)

C Chronic health points:

If the patient has a history of severe organ system insufficiency or is immunocompromised assign points as follows:

1 For non-operative or emergency post-operative patients. 5 points.

2 For elective post-operative patients. 2 points.

Definitions

Organ insufficiency or immunocompromised state must have been evident prior to this hospital admission and conform to the following criteria:

Liver: Biopsy proven cirrhosis and documented portal hypertension; episodes of past upper GI bleeding attributed to portal hypertension or prior episodes of hepatic failure/encephalopathy/coma.

Cardiovascular: New York Heart Association Class IV.

Respiratory: Chronic restrictive, obstructive or vascular disease resulting in severe exercise restriction. i.e. unable to climb stairs or perform household duties, or documented chronic hypoxia, hypercapnia, secondary polycythaemia, severe pulmonary hypertension (>40 mmHg) or respiratory dependency.

Immunocompromised: The patient has received therapy that suppresses resistance to infection. e.g. immunosuppression, chemotherapy, radiation, long-term or recent high dose steroids, or has a disease that is sufficiently advanced to suppress resistance to infection. e.g. leukaemia, lymphoma, AIDS.

APACHE II score

Sum of **A** + **B** + **C**

A APS points _____

B Age points _____

C Chronic health points _____

Total APACHE II _____

5.5 Diagnosis of brain death in the United Kingdom

The development of techniques for resuscitation of the cardiovascular system and artificial support of respiration has led inevitably to the problem of some patients being maintained on a mechanical ventilator with a beating heart when the brain is irretrievably dead.

It is now generally agreed that death of the brain and brain stem function is an indication to withdraw all artificial support. With this in mind the Medical Royal Colleges drew up a joint statement in which they defined a number of conditions that should be satisfied, in order that all forms of support can be withdrawn in the sure knowledge that recovery is no longer possible.

This report was published in full in *British Medical Journal* (1976) **2**, 1187–1188 and the conditions and tests recommended in that report are summarized below.

5.5.1 Conditions for considering brain death

All the following should coexist:
1 The patient is deeply comatose.
   a Exclude the presence of cerebral depressant drugs, particularly if hypothermia is present or there is a history of drug ingestion.
   b Exclude hypothermia, body temperature should be at least 35°C.
   c Exclude abnormalities of metabolism or endocrine system. In particular abnormalities of serum electrolytes, acid base balance, blood sugar.
2 The patient is being maintained on a ventilator because spontaneous respiration had previously become inadequate or had ceased altogether. Exclude presence of muscle relaxant drugs or other respiratory depressants.
3 There should be no doubt that the patient's condition is due to irremediable structural brain damage. The diagnosis of a disorder which can lead to brain death should have been fully established.

5.5.2 Tests for confirming brain death

All brain stem reflexes should be absent.
1 The pupils are fixed in diameter and do not respond to sharp changes in the intensity of incident light.

2 There is no corneal reflex.

3 The vestibuloocular reflexes are absent. These are absent when no eye movement occurs during or after the slow injection of 20 ml of ice-cold water into each auditory meatus in turn. Clear access to the tympanic membrane must have been established by direct inspection. This test may be contraindicated by local trauma.

4 No motor responses within the cranial nerve distribution can be elicited by adequate stimulation of any somatic area.

5 There is no gag reflex or reflex response to bronchial stimulation by a suction catheter passed down the trachea.

6 No respiratory movements occur when the patient is disconnected from the mechanical ventilator long enough to ensure that P_{CO_2} rises above 6.7 kPa. Blood gases should be measured and recorded. Patients with pre-existing chronic respiratory disease, may be unresponsive to raised P_{CO_2} and exist on a hypoxic drive to respiration. These cases must be carefully evaluated with blood gas measurements.

5.5.3 Recommended procedure

1 Pre-oxygenate with 100% oxygen for 5 minutes.

2 Take and record arterial blood gas sample.

3 Disconnect patient from the ventilator for up to 6 min to enable the P_aCO_2 to rise to at least 6.7 kPa (50 mmHg). Maintain oxygenation by insufflation of oxygen at 8 l/min.

4 Take and record arterial blood gas sample.

As an alternative the P_aCO_2 can be raised to the required level by pre-ventilation with 5% carbon dioxide in oxygen before the ventilator is disconnected.

5.5.4 Other considerations

Integrity of spinal reflexes
Spinal reflexes can persist after irretrievable destruction of brain stem function, and may be present in brain dead patients.

Confirmatory investigations
Electroencephalography, cerebral angiography or cerebral blood flow measurements are not necessary to diagnose brain death.

Body temperature
Must be above 35 C before tests are carried out.

Specialist opinion and status of doctors concerned
The diagnosis of brain death should be made by two medical practitioners who have expertise in this field. Clinicians with wide experience of intensive therapy or acute medicine should not need specialist advice, but if there is any doubt it is necessary to consult a neurologist or neurosurgeon.

One of the two must be a consultant, the other a consultant or senior registrar who should assure themselves that the preconditions have been met before testing is carried out. The length of time required before preconditions can be satisfied varies according to circumstances, and although occasionally it might be less than 24 hours, it may extend to several days.

The two doctors may carry out the tests separately or together. If the tests confirm brain death they should nevertheless be repeated.

There may be circumstances in which it is impossible or inappropriate to carry out every one of the tests. The criteria published by the conference give recommended guidelines rather than rigid rules and it is for the doctors at the bedside to decide when the patient is dead.

Repetition of testing
It is customary to repeat the tests to ensure that there has been no observer error. The interval between tests varies with the diagnosis and clinical course of the disease. It is common in practice to allow 24 hours to elapse, but this interval might be very much less and no particular time is suggested in the statement.

It is for the two doctors to decide how long the interval between tests should be but the time should be adequate for the reassurance of all those directly concerned. At the conclusion of each set of tests, each doctor must record their findings on the form that is available in all hospitals in the UK. This record must be attached to the patient's notes.

5.6 Transplantation checklist

If a patient who has been certified brain dead is to be considered for organ donation the following points must be considered and noted:

1 Brain death must be confirmed by two consultants or a consultant and senior registrar appropriately qualified to do so. Above all they must be completely independent of the transplant team.

2 There must be no reason to believe that the patient would have objected to the organ donation, and that even when express permission has been granted, the views of the relatives are given due consideration. The necessity to remove organs immediately after death is not sufficient reason to make such enquiries impracticable.

3 Authorization to proceed with transplantation must also be obtained from whoever is in lawful possession of the body. When a person dies in hospital, this would be the health authority, represented by the unit general manager.

4 If the death would, in normal circumstances, be reported to the coroner, his permission must be obtained before transplantation can proceed.

5 The local transplant coordinator should be contacted as soon as possible.

Telephone number of local transplant coordinator . . . .

The transplant team will decide ultimately if the donor is a suitable source of organs; the following basic information will be of help in this decision:

Age

Cause of death

Results of recent haematology, biochemistry, and liver function tests

Blood group

Status of circulation, respiratory function, renal function and liver.

Absence of local or systemic infection, malignancy (other than primary brain tumour) and other disease relevant to the organ donation

If not already tested the following investigations will be necessary:
Hepatitis B antigen
Human immunosuppressive virus (HIV)
Tissue typing

5

Section 6
The Cardiovascular System

6

6.1 ECG times

6.1.1 Normal ECG times

P wave	Atrial wave	<0.10 s
PR interval	Atrioventricular conduction	$0.12–0.20$ s
QRS time	Rapid ventricular depolarization	$0.05–0.08$ s
QT time	Length of ventricular complex	$0.35–0.40$ s
T wave	Repolarization	≤ 0.22 s

6.1.2 Calculating rate/min from the ECG trace at 25 mm/s

Small squares $= 0.04$ s
Large squares $= 0.2$ s
i.e. 5 small squares $= 1$ large square

6

If 1 large square lies between R waves $=$ rate of 300/min
   2 large squares lie between R waves $=$ rate of 150/min
   3 large squares lie between R waves $=$ rate of 100/min
   4 large squares lie between R waves $=$ rate of 75/min
   5 large squares lie between R waves $=$ rate of 60/min
i.e. 300 divided by number of large squares between R
waves $=$ pulse rate.

6.2 Arrhythmias and abnormal ECG patterns

Sinus bradycardia

Usually between 40–60 beats/min. PR interval increased, QT interval increased.

Clinical significance. Can be normal (sleep) or due to high vagal tone.

Treatment. Usually none. If symptomatic, atropine 0.6–1 mg i.v. or consider pacing.

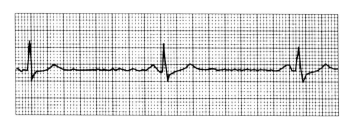

Atrial fibrillation

Atrial rate if visible 400–700 beats/min, ventricular rate irregular often fast, up to 200 beats/min.

Clinical significance. Usually indicates heart disease.

Treatment. Patients with longstanding atrial fibrillation secondary to cardiac disease will usually be on digoxin. Acute atrial fibrillation can be treated by:

1 Verapamil 5–10 mg i.v. slowly. This drug should be used with extreme caution if the patient is already taking beta blocking drugs.
2 Disopyramide: 100 mg or 2 mg/kg (max. 150 mg) i.v. over 5 minutes.
3 Flecainide: 2 mg/kg i.v. over 20 minutes (max. 150 mg)
4 Digoxin: three doses of 0.5 mg i.v. through a burette over 30, 60 and 120 minutes in the first 24 h. Oral maintenance dose 0.25 mg daily.
5 DC shock.

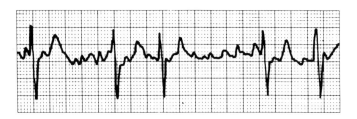

Atrial flutter

Atrial rate 200–400 beats/min with 2:1, 3:1, or 4:1 ventricular response. Ventricular rate thus 100–150 beats/min. Flutter (F) waves usually visible.

Clinical significance. Ventricular rate needs to be controlled.

Treatment. As follows:

1 Verapamil 5–10 mg i.v. (and repeat if necessary).
2 Consider disopyramide.
3 Consider flecainide.
4 Consider amiodarone.
5 Consider propanolol.
6 Consider DC shock.

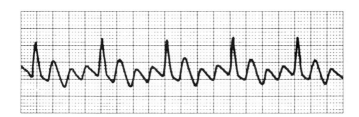

First degree atrioventricular block

PR interval greater than 0.20 s.

Clinical significance. Frequently none.

Treatment. None.

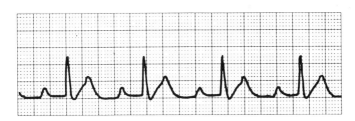

Second degree atrioventricular block

1 Wenckebach block (illustrated below). PR interval increasing until a ventricular complex is dropped.

Clinical significance. Variable, may be seen in normal people during sleep or after acute myocardial infarction.

Treatment. Usually none unless symptomatic.

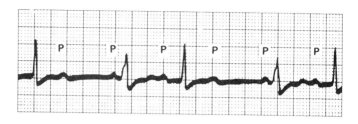

2 Mobitz block. PR interval prolonged. Intermittent dropped ventricular beat. Usually associated with wide QRS complex.
Clinical significance. May forewarn of sudden complete atrioventricular (AV) dissociation.
Treatment. Usually requires cardiac pacing.

Third degree block
P waves are regular and of normal rate but are dissociated from the ventricular complexes. The ventricular rate is usually slow.
1 Narrow complex ventricular rhythm.
Clinical significance. May be congenital or acquired. Treat if symptomatic.
2 Wide complex ventricular rhythm.
Clinical significance. Usually requires pacing. May indicate a poor prognosis.

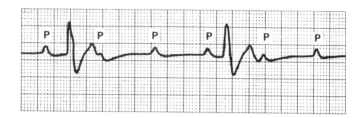

Left bundle branch block
Seen in leads V_1 or V_6. The broad-notched QRS complexes and deformed ST segments are individually reminiscent of ventricular ectopic complexes.

Clinical significance. May lead to a third degree atrioventricular block if associated with acute ischaemic heart disease. As seen in V$_6$ or Lead I the QRS is wide (120 ms) with T wave in opposite direction.

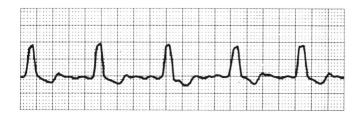

Right bundle branch block

As seen in V$_1$ a typical RSR pattern is shown here with normal sinus rhythm. When these bizarre, wide repetitive QRS complexes do not follow obvious P waves, they can be difficult to distinguish from those of ventricular tachycardia.

Clinical significance. May occasionally herald AV block if it follows cardiac infarction.

Treatment. Usually none, but if RBBB is associated with ECG evidence of left or right axis deviation and a long P–R interval, insertion of a temporary pacemaker should be considered.

6

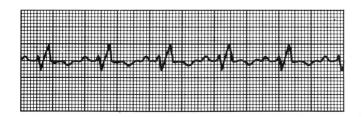

Pacemaker rhythm

It is common to see the pacing impulse just before a QRS
complex, but the pacing spike may be absent. P waves may
occasionally be observed.

Clinical significance. Indicates satisfactory capture of the heart by
the pacemaker. When used in the demand mode, the pacemaker
may have some or all complexes suppressed by the patient's
spontaneous complexes.

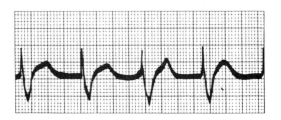

Atrial extrasystole

A P wave usually followed by a QRS complex causes an irregular
rhythm. Atrial systoles may be non-conducted (not followed by a
QRS complex), conducted normally or with a prolonged PR
interval.

Clinical significance. Essentially benign. May herald atrial
tachycardia, flutter or fibrillation (AF).

Treatment. None.

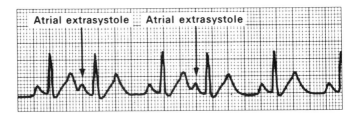

Supraventricular tachycardia

QRS with fast rate and P waves visible or within the QRS complex.

Clinical significance. May revert spontaneously, but if prolonged or if cardiac output is compromised treatment is necessary.

Treatment. As follows:

1 Carotid sinus pressure or Valsalva manoeuvre.

2 Verapamil 10 mg i.v. This dose can be repeated after an interval if necessary, with frequent blood pressure monitoring.

3 Consider DC shock, particularly if the patient's general condition deteriorates.

4 Consider flecainide.

5 Consider amiodarone.

6 Consider beta blocker (propanolol).

6

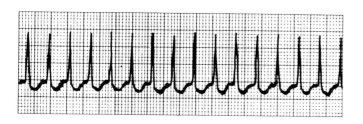

Ventricular extrasystoles

Abnormal ventricular extra beat occurs often, with abnormal T wave. No P wave precedes the abnormal beat.

Clinical significance. May sometimes precede ventricular tachycardia (VT) or ventricular fibrillation (VF).

Treatment. The decision whether to treat or to ignore ventricular extrasystoles depends on individual circumstances. These include the frequency of the abnormal beats, their aetiology and the patient's general condition. Possible treatments include the following:

1 Lignocaine 100 mg i.v. If this is successful, it should be followed by a lignocaine infusion starting at 3 mg/min.

2 Check—plasma potassium, blood sugar, blood gases and acid base balance. Digoxin may be an aetiological factor. Myocardial irritation may be caused by a central venous pressure line, Swan–Ganz catheter, or a mediastinal drain.

3 Consider amiodarone.

4 Consider disopyramide.

5 Consider beta blocker.

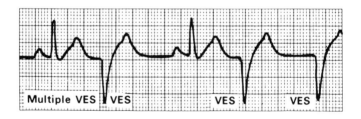

Ventricular tachycardia

Regular fast rhythm with abnormal ventricular complexes. Wide notch QRS complexes frequently seen. Rate usually 140–280 beats/min.

Clinical significance. Potentially dangerous except for 'slow' forms. High risk of transition to VF.

1 Lignocaine 100 mg i.v. followed by an infusion at 3 mg/min.
2 Consider flecainide.
3 Consider amiodarone.
4 Consider disopyramide.
5 If treatment not immediately successful or the patient's condition deteriorates, immediate DC shock.

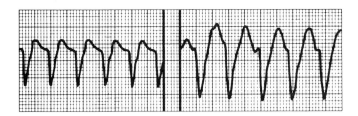

6

Ventricular fibrillation

Chaotic irregular ventricular pattern.
Clinical significance. Circulatory arrest.
Treatment. External cardiac massage and DC shock.

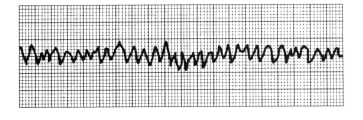

Summary of doses of antidysrhythmic drugs mentioned in this section

Drug	Loading dose i.v.	Oral dose
Amiodarone	5 mg/kg infusion over 20 min to 2 h, then up to 1200 mg over 24 h	200 mg t.d.s.
Digoxin	Three doses of 0.5 mg i.v. Infuse through burette over 30, 60 and 120 min in first 24 h	0.125–0.25 mg D
Disopyramide	2 mg/kg over 5 min (max. 150 mg). 400 µg/kg/h by infusion (max. 800 mg D)	300–800 mg daily DD
Flecainide	2 mg/kg in 10–30 min (max. 150 mg). Infusion 1.5 mg/kg/h for 1 h, then 0.25 mg/kg/h	100–200 mg b.d.
Lignocaine	100 mg i.v. Start infusion at 3 mg/min and then reduce	
Propanolol	1 mg i.v. Repeat up to max. 10 mg	10–40 mg t.d.s.
Verapamil	5–10 mg i.v.	40–120 mg t.d.s.

6.3 Cardiac data

6.3.1 Distribution of cardiac output to body organs

	Average wt (kg)	% body wt	Blood flow (ml/min)	% cardiac output	O_2 consumption (ml/min/organ)
Brain	1.4	2.0	775	15	46
Heart	0.3	0.43	175	3.3	23
Kidneys	0.3	0.43	1100	23	18
Liver	1.5	2.1	1400	29	66
Lungs	1.0	1.5	175	3.5	5
Muscle	27.8	39.7	1000	19	64
Rest	38.7	55.34	375	9.7	33

6.3.2 Cardiovascular pressures

	Systolic (mmHg)	Diastolic (mmHg)	Mean (mmHg)
Peripheral venous			6–12
Right atrium (CVP)			0–7
Right ventricle	14–32	0–7	12–17
Pulmonary artery	14–32	2–13	8–19
Wedge or left atrium			6–12
Left ventricle	100–150	2–12	
Arterial	100–150	60–90	80–100

6

6.4 Dosage of drugs delivered by infusion

The two tables following indicate the dose of drugs diluted and delivered by infusion through three sizes of drip set. The dose is shown in μg/min and in μg/kg/min calculated for 50, 70 and 90 kg.

The doses shown are for two dilutions, 20 μg/ml and 500 μg/ml, with examples of how these dilutions might be achieved. Other drip rates and concentrations can easily be calculated from these basic tables.

Concentration: 2 mg in 100 ml or 10 mg in 500 ml = 20 μg/ml

| | Drip set 15 drops/ml | | | | Drip set 20 drops/ml | | | | Drip set 60 drops/ml | | | |
| | | μg/kg/min | | | | μg/kg/min | | | | μg/kg/min | | |
Drops/min	μg/min	50 kg	70 kg	90 kg	μg/min	50 kg	70 kg	90 kg	μg/min	50 kg	70 kg	90 kg
1	1.3	0.03	0.02	0.01	1	0.02	0.014	0.011	0.3	0.007	0.005	0.004
2	2.7	0.05	0.04	0.03	2	0.04	0.03	0.02	0.7	0.01	0.009	0.007
3	4	0.08	0.06	0.04	3	0.06	0.04	0.03	1	0.02	0.014	0.01
4	5.3	0.1	0.08	0.06	4	0.08	0.06	0.04	1.3	0.03	0.02	0.015
5	6.7	0.13	0.01	0.07	5	0.1	0.07	0.05	1.7	0.033	0.024	0.018
10	13	0.3	0.2	0.1	10	0.2	0.14	0.11	3.3	0.07	0.05	0.04
20	27	0.5	0.4	0.3	20	0.4	0.3	0.2	6.7	0.13	0.1	0.07
30	40	0.8	0.6	0.4	30	0.6	0.4	0.3	10	0.2	0.14	0.11
40	53	1.1	0.8	0.6	40	0.8	0.6	0.4	13	0.3	0.19	0.15
50	67	1.3	0.9	0.7	50	1	0.7	0.5	17	0.3	0.24	0.18
60	80	1.6	1.1	0.9	60	1.2	0.9	0.7	20	0.4	0.28	0.2
70	93	1.9	1.3	1	70	1.4	1	0.8	23	0.5	0.33	0.26
80	107	2.1	1.5	1.2	80	1.6	1.1	0.9	27	0.53	0.38	0.3
90	120	2.4	1.7	1.3	90	1.8	1.3	1	30	0.6	0.43	0.33
100	133	2.7	1.9	1.5	100	2	1.4	1.1	33	0.7	0.47	0.37

Concentration: 50 mg in 100 ml or 250 mg in 500 ml = 500 µg/ml

1	33	0.7	0.5	0.4	25	0.5	0.4	0.3	8.3	0.2	0.12	0.1
2	67	1.3	1	0.7	50	1	0.7	0.5	17	0.3	0.2	0.18
3	100	2	1.4	1.1	75	1.5	1.1	0.8	25	0.5	0.4	0.3
4	133	2.7	1.9	1.5	100	2	1.4	1.1	33	0.7	0.5	0.4
5	167	3.3	2.4	1.8	125	2.5	1.8	1.4	42	0.8	0.6	0.5
10	333	6.7	4.8	3.7	250	5	3.6	2.8	83	1.7	1.2	0.9
20	667	13	9.5	7.4	500	10	7.1	5.5	167	3.3	2.4	1.9
30	1000	20	14	11	750	15	11	8.3	250	5	3.6	2.8
40	1333	27	19	15	1000	20	14	11	333	6.7	4.8	3.7
50	1667	33	24	19	1250	25	18	14	417	8.3	5.9	4.6
60	2000	40	29	22	1500	30	21	17	500	10	7.1	5.5
70	2333	47	33	26	1750	35	25	19	583	12	8.3	6.5
80	2667	53	38	30	2000	40	29	22	667	13	9.5	7.4
90	3000	60	43	33	2250	45	32	25	750	15	11	8.3
100	3333	67	48	37	2500	50	36	28	833	17	12	9.3

6

6.5 Dilution and administration of common drugs acting on the cardiovascular and respiratory systems

1 All drugs can be diluted in 5% dextrose; for other possible diluents see manufacturer's data sheet.

2 Glyceryl trinitrate and isosorbide are incompatible with PVC containers or drip sets. Glass, polyethylene or polybutadiene can be used.

3 Always infuse using a drip counter or syringe pump.

4 In an intensive therapy unit, higher concentrations than those shown can be used if higher doses or fluid restriction is necessary.

5 The suggested starting doses are only a guideline. The dose of a drug required is ultimately dependent on clinical response, and may therefore need to be adjusted rapidly up or down.

6 All these drugs must only be used by medical and nursing staff who understand the pharmacology involved and are prepared to monitor the patient very closely.

7 The use of 100 ml as a diluting volume is often to be preferred in the interest of economy. The drug is diluted in a 100 ml burette delivering 1 ml per 60 drops. The higher concentrations are another reason to ensure safety with a drip counter.

Drug	Dilution	Concentration	Starting dose (70 kg)	
			ml/h	µg/kg/min
Adrenaline	2 mg in 100 ml	20 µg/ml	15	0.07
Aminophylline	500 mg in 100 ml	5 mg/ml	17	20
	500 mg in 500 ml	1 mg/ml	83	20
Dobutamine*	250 mg in 100 ml	2.5 mg/ml	10	6
Dopamine*	200 mg in 100 ml	2 mg/ml	7	3.3
Glyceryl trinitrate	50 mg in 50 ml	1 mg/ml	4	0.95
Isoprenaline	1 mg in 100 ml	10 µg/ml	20	0.05
Isosorbide	50 mg in 100 ml	0.5 mg/ml	4	0.5
Labetalol	100 mg in 100 ml	1 mg/ml	20	4.8
Lignocaine	1 g in 500 ml	2 mg/ml	60	28
	2 g in 500 ml	4 mg/ml	30	28
Nitroprusside	50 mg in 100 ml	500 µg/ml	5	0.6
	50 mg in 250 ml	200 µg/ml	4.5	0.2

Note: Higher concentrations are commonly used after cardiac surgery when rapid control is necessary. Max. recommended dose: 400 µg/min (6 µg/kg/min)

Drug	Dilution	Concentration	ml/h	µg/kg/min
Noradrenaline	2 mg in 100 ml	20 µg/ml	15	0.07
Salbutamol	5 mg in 500 ml	10 µg/ml	30	0.07

* *Alternative dilution for dobutamine and dopamine:*
   1 Multiply patient body weight by six.
   2 Dissolve the resultant figure in mg in 100 ml of diluent.
   3 When this solution is infused the ml infused per hour = µg/kg/min.

Section 7
Lung Function

7

7.1 Ventilatory abbreviations

These abbreviations are suitably divided into primary symbols, written in capitals, and secondary symbols, written in capitals or lower case in the inferior position typographically.

7.1.1 Primary symbols

C concentration of gas in blood phase
D diffusing capacity
F fractional concentration in the dry gas phase
P gas pressure, i.e. partial pressure
Q volume of blood
R respiratory exchange ratio
S saturation of haemoglobin with oxygen or carbon dioxide
V gas volume

7.1.2 Secondary symbols

A alveolar gas
a arterial gas
B barometric
c pulmonary capillary blood
D dead space gas
E expired gas
I inspired gas
T tidal gas
v venous blood

A dash above a symbol indicates the mean value, e.g. $\bar{V}$ = mean volume of gas. A dot above a symbol indicates per unit time, e.g. $\dot{V}$ = volume of gas per unit time.

STPD = standard temperature and pressure dry
BTPS = body temperature and pressure saturated with water vapour
ATPS = ambient temperature and pressure saturated with water vapour

Examples
$P_A CO_2$ = partial pressure of carbon dioxide in alveolar gas
$\dot{Q}$ = volume of blood per unit time, or cardiac output
$F_I O_2$ = fractional concentration of inspired oxygen
P_B = barometric pressure

7.2 Respiratory and ventilatory parameters (adult)

Airways resistance	1.6 cm H_2O/l/sec
Alveolar ventilation	4.2 l/min
Carbon dioxide production	150–200 ml/min
Compliance of chest wall and lung	0.1 l/cm H_2O
Compliance of chest wall	0.2 l/cm H_2O
Compliance of lung	0.2 l/cm H_2O
Dead space	150 ml
Diffusion capacity of carbon monoxide	17–20 ml CO/min/mmHg
Expiratory reserve volume	950–1200 ml
Forced expiratory volume 1 second	75% vital capacity
Fractional carbon monoxide uptake	53%
Functional residual capacity	2300–2800 ml
Inspiratory capacity	3600–4300 ml
Inspiratory reserve volume	3300–3750 ml
Lung segments on left	5 + 3
Lung segments on right	3 + 2 + 4
Lung weight	80 g
Max. ventilatory volume	120 l/min
Minute volume	5000–6000 ml/min
Number of airways	14 × 1 000 000
Number of alveoli	296 × 1 000 000
Oxygen availability in normal lungs	950–1050 ml/min
Oxygen consumption	200–250 ml/min
Peak expiratory flow rate	400 l/min
Peak inspiratory flow rate	300 l/min
Pulmonary capillary blood flow	5400 ml/min
Pulmonary capillary blood volume	60 ml
Pulmonary capillary pressure	8 mmHg (1.07 kPa)
Residual volume	1200–1700 ml
Respiratory quotient	0.8 on normal diet
Respiratory rate	12–14/min
Tidal volume	400–600 ml
Total lung capacity	5000–6500 ml
Vital capacity	4200–4800 ml
Work of breathing (max.)	98 J/min
Work of breathing (normal)	4.9 J/min

7.3 Lung volumes and capacities

Given as a percentage of total lung capacity, an average of 6000 ml for an adult, down to 900 ml for a 10 kg child.

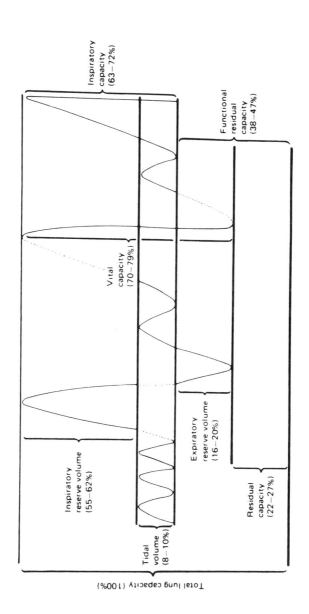

7

7.4 Pulmonary function tables

7.4.1 Peak expiratory flow rate prediction table (l/min)

Height			Age (years)					
cm	ft	in	20	25	30	35	40	45
Males								
160	5	3	572	572	560	548	536	524
168	5	6	597	597	584	572	559	547
175	5	9	625	625	612	599	586	573
183	6	0	654	654	640	626	613	599
191	6	3	679	679	665	650	636	622
Females								
145	4	9	377	377	366	356	345	335
152	5	0	403	403	392	382	371	361
160	5	3	433	433	422	412	401	391
168	5	6	459	459	448	438	427	417
175	5	9	489	489	478	468	457	447

Height			Age (years)					
cm	ft	in	50	55	60	65	70	75
Males								
160	5	3	512	500	488	476	464	452
168	5	6	534	522	509	496	484	472
175	5	9	560	547	533	520	507	494
183	6	0	585	572	558	544	530	516
191	6	3	608	593	579	565	551	537
Females								
145	4	9	324	314	303	293	282	272
152	5	0	350	340	329	319	308	298
160	5	3	380	370	359	349	338	328
168	5	6	406	396	385	375	364	354
175	5	9	436	426	415	405	394	384

One standard deviation = 60 l/min.

7.4.2 Vitalograph

A good picture of respiratory function can be obtained from this graph. If successive tests are performed, this will give an indication of the progress of the lung disease and its treatment.

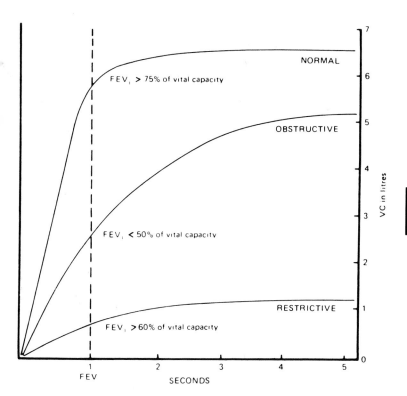

In obstructive lung disease the slope of the graph is depressed.
In restrictive lung disease the ultimate vital capacity is reduced.

7.4.3 Forced vital capacity prediction table (litres)

Height			Age (years)					
cm	ft	in	20	25	30	35	40	45
Males								
160	5	3	4.17	4.17	4.06	3.95	3.84	3.73
168	5	6	4.53	4.53	4.42	4.31	4.20	4.09
175	5	9	4.95	4.95	4.84	4.73	4.62	4.51
183	6	0	5.37	5.37	5.26	5.15	5.04	4.93
191	6	3	5.73	5.73	5.62	5.51	5.40	5.29
Females								
145	4	9	3.13	3.13	2.98	2.83	2.68	2.53
152	5	0	3.45	3.45	3.30	3.15	3.00	2.85
160	5	3	3.83	3.83	3.68	3.53	3.38	3.23
168	5	6	4.20	4.20	4.05	3.90	3.75	3.60
175	5	9	4.53	4.53	4.38	4.23	4.08	3.93

Height			Age (years)					
cm	ft	in	50	55	60	65	70	75
Males								
160	5	3	3.62	3.51	3.40	3.29	3.18	3.07
168	5	6	3.98	3.87	3.76	3.65	3.54	3.43
175	5	9	4.40	4.29	4.18	4.07	3.96	3.85
183	6	0	4.82	4.71	4.60	4.49	4.38	4.27
191	6	3	5.18	5.07	4.96	4.85	4.74	4.63
Females								
145	4	9	2.38	2.23	2.08	1.93	1.78	1.63
152	5	0	2.70	2.55	2.40	2.25	2.10	1.95
160	5	3	3.08	2.93	2.78	2.63	2.48	2.33
168	5	6	3.45	3.30	3.15	3.00	2.85	2.70
175	5	9	3.78	3.63	3.48	3.33	3.18	3.03

Males: one standard deviation = 0.6 litres.
Females: one standard deviation = 0.4 litres.

7.4.4 Vital capacity in children

Boys: 4–9   years = (193 × age in years) + 88
         10–12 years = (194 × age in years) + 83
Girls: 4–11 years = (191 × age in years) − 62
         12–16 years = (200 × age in years) − 121

7.4.5 Forced expiratory volume prediction table (at 1 second in litres)

Height			Age (years)					
cm	ft	in	20	25	30	35	40	45
Males								
160	5	3	3.61	3.61	3.45	3.30	3.14	2.99
168	5	6	3.86	3.86	3.71	3.55	3.40	3.24
175	5	9	4.15	4.15	4	3.84	3.69	3.53
183	6	0	4.44	4.44	4.28	4.13	3.97	3.82
191	6	3	4.69	4.69	4.54	4.38	4.23	4.07
Females								
145	4	9	2.60	2.60	2.45	2.30	2.15	2
152	5	0	2.83	2.83	2.68	2.53	2.38	2.23
160	5	3	3.09	3.09	2.94	2.79	2.64	2.49
168	5	6	3.36	3.36	3.21	3.06	2.91	2.76
175	5	9	3.59	3.59	3.44	3.29	3.14	2.99

Height			Age (years)					
cm	ft	in	50	55	60	65	70	75
Males								
160	5	3	2.83	2.68	2.52	2.37	2.21	2.06
168	5	6	3.09	2.93	2.78	2.62	2.47	2.31
175	5	9	3.38	3.22	3.06	2.91	2.75	2.60
183	6	0	3.66	3.51	3.35	3.20	3.04	2.89
191	6	3	3.92	3.76	3.61	3.45	3.30	3.14
Females								
145	4	9	1.85	1.70	1.55	1.40	1.25	1.10
152	5	0	2.08	1.93	1.78	1.63	1.48	1.33
160	5	3	2.34	2.19	2.04	1.89	1.74	1.59
168	5	6	2.61	2.46	2.31	2.16	2.01	1.86
175	5	9	2.84	2.69	2.54	2.39	2.24	2.09

7

Males: one standard deviation = 0.5 litres
Females: one standard deviation = 0.4 litres

7.5 Gases (at P_B 760 mmHg or 101.1 kPa)

7.5.1 Normal partial pressure of gases

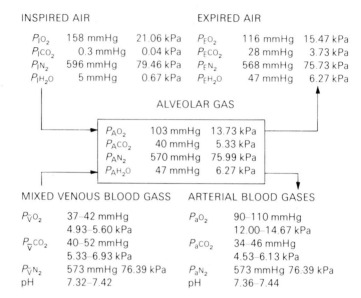

INSPIRED AIR

P_IO_2	158 mmHg	21.06 kPa
P_ICO_2	0.3 mmHg	0.04 kPa
P_IN_2	596 mmHg	79.46 kPa
P_IH_2O	5 mmHg	0.67 kPa

EXPIRED AIR

P_EO_2	116 mmHg	15.47 kPa
P_ECO_2	28 mmHg	3.73 kPa
P_EN_2	568 mmHg	75.73 kPa
P_EH_2O	47 mmHg	6.27 kPa

ALVEOLAR GAS

P_AO_2	103 mmHg	13.73 kPa
P_ACO_2	40 mmHg	5.33 kPa
P_AN_2	570 mmHg	75.99 kPa
P_AH_2O	47 mmHg	6.27 kPa

MIXED VENOUS BLOOD GASS

$P_{\bar{V}}O_2$	37–42 mmHg
	4.93–5.60 kPa
$P_{\bar{V}}CO_2$	40–52 mmHg
	5.33–6.93 kPa
$P_{\bar{V}}N_2$	573 mmHg 76.39 kPa
pH	7.32–7.42

ARTERIAL BLOOD GASES

P_aO_2	90–110 mmHg
	12.00–14.67 kPa
P_aCO_2	34–46 mmHg
	4.53–6.13 kPa
P_aN_2	573 mmHg 76.39 kPa
pH	7.36–7.44

7.5.2 Normal content of gases

Inspired: C_IO_2 20.93%
$\quad\quad\quad$ C_ICO_2 0.03%
Mixed venous: $C_{\bar{V}}O_2$ 15%
$\quad\quad\quad\quad$ $C_{\bar{V}}CO_2$ 52%
Arterial: C_aO_2 20–21%
$\quad\quad\quad$ C_aCO_2 48–50%

7.5.3 Oxygen availability to tissues

$$\left[\frac{Hb(g/dl) \times 1.34 \times sat.\ O_2}{100} + 0.0225 \times P_aO_2\ (kPa) \right] \times$$

$$\times\ cardiac\ output\ (ml)$$

(1.34 = the amount of O_2 transported per g of Hb;
$0.0225 \times P_aO_2$ (kPa) = the amount of O_2 dissolved in plasma)

$$\text{Normally} = \left[\frac{14 \times 1.34 \times 98}{100} + 0.0225 \times 14 \right] \times \frac{5000}{100}$$

$$\simeq 950\text{--}1000 \text{ ml/min}$$

The brain cannot extract O_2 below a lower limit of availability of 450 ml/min.

7.6 Ventilation equations

7.6.1 Alveolar air equation

$$P_AO_2 = P_IO_2 - \frac{P_ACO_2}{RQ} = 100 \text{ mmHg}$$

(RQ depends on diet—normally 0.8)

An easy method of working out shunt and venous dead space equations is shown below.

7.6.2 Dead space equation

$$\frac{V_D}{V_T} = \frac{P_ACO_2 - P_ECO_2}{P_ACO_2} = 0.3$$

P_ACO_2 is calculated from the alveolar air equation (7.6.1) (usually taken as the same as P_aCO_2).

$\quad P_ECO_2$ is collected and measured by Campbell's modification of the Haldane apparatus.

7.6.3 Percentage venous admixture equation (or shunt equation)

$$\frac{\dot{Q}_S}{\dot{Q}_T} = \frac{C_cO_2 - C_aO_2}{C_cO_2 - C_{\bar{V}}O_2} = 5\% \text{ of cardiac output}$$

$\dot{Q}_T$ = total flow through lungs; $\dot{Q}_S$ = flow through shunt.

C_cO_2 is measured from the alveolar air equation, it is assumed that $C_cO_2 \equiv C_AO_2$.

C_aO_2: take arterial and venous blood gases and convert to C_VO_2 percentage content.

7.6.4. Alveolar–arterial oxygen difference

$P_{A}O_2 - P_{a}O_2 = $ 5–20 mmHg breathing air (0.66–2.66 kPa)
$= $ 10–60 mmHg breathing 100% O_2 (1.3–7.99 kPa)

If the alveolar–arterial difference is 120–300 mmHg
(15.9–39.9 kPa) when breathing 100% O_2 then the patient needs
40% O_2 added by mask to maintain arterial Po_2. If it is 350
(46.6 kPa) on 100% O_2 then the patient probably has such a large
shunt that this cannot be corrected without assisted ventilation.

Alternatively, if the patient has an alveolar–arterial difference of
250 (33.3 kPa) when breathing 50% O_2, then ventilation is
probably necessary.

7.6.5 Po_2 reduction with age

The older the patient, the lower the normal $P_{a}O_2$. The formula
below indicates the expected $P_{a}O_2$ of patients pre-and post-op.

$$\text{Pre-op. fit patient} = 104 - \frac{\text{age}}{4} \text{ mmHg} (\times 0.133 \text{ kPa})$$

$$\text{Post-op. 24–36 h} = 94 - \frac{\text{age}}{2} \text{ mmHg} (\times 0.133 \text{ kPa})$$

7.6.6 Respiratory quotient

Oxygen consumption   = 200–250 ml per min
Carbon dioxide production = 150–200 ml per min

$$\text{Respiratory quotient} = \frac{CO_2 \text{ produced}}{O_2 \text{ consumed}} = 0.8 \text{ on a normal diet}$$

7.7 **Virtual shunt lines**

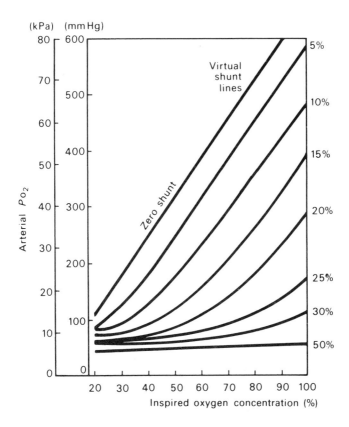

Mean values for arterial Po_2 plotted against inspired oxygen
concentrations for 15 published studies of anaesthetized patients

Shunt calculation

To calculate shunt, read off $F_{I}O_2\%$ (inspired oxygen concentration)
on an air/oxygen mixing chart. Obtain P_aO_2 from arterial blood gas
analysis. The percentage shunt can then be determined by using
the virtual shunt lines.

7.8 Added oxygen to ventilator nomogram

Relating the minute volume, added oxygen and oxygen percentage of resulting mixture. Fix the minute volume and the required O_2 percentage. The O_2 (l/min) to be added is shown in the middle line.

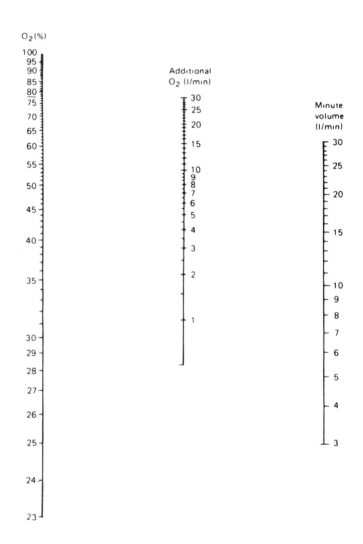

7.9 Inspired oxygen to atmospheric pressure nomogram

Relating atmospheric pressure, oxygen percentage and inspired oxygen tension. From the atmospheric pressure and the O_2 concentration percentage, the P_1O_2 can be found.

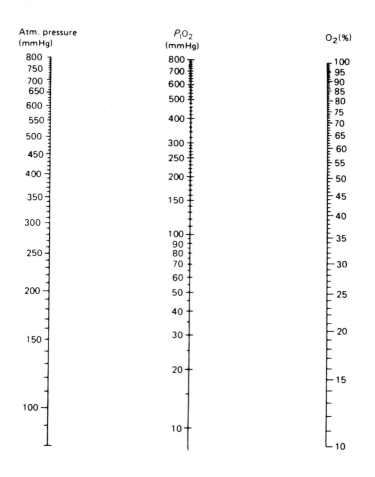

Section 8
Renal Failure

8

8.1 Diagnosis of renal failure

Urine	Renal	Prerenal	Normal
Osmolality	285–295	<400	400–1400
Response to Lasix 500 mg	Poor	Fair	Very good
Blood/urine urea ratio	<5:1	<10:1	20:1 or more
Urine/plasma osmality ratio	<1:1	1:1–2	2:1 or more
Creatinine	<120	<120	45–100 mmol/24 h
Sodium	>20	<10 mmol/l	

8.2 Management of acute renal failure

Renal failure occurs when renal function is inadequate to control electrolyte and fluid balance. Acute renal failure progresses rapidly over a few hours or days and is characterized by rapid rises in blood urea (normal range 2.6–6.5 mmol/l), creatinine (normal range 45–120 μmol/l) and potassium (normal range 3.8–5 mmol/l). Oliguria commonly occurs (500 ml urine in 24 hours), but acute renal failure can also be present with normal or increased urine volumes.

8

8.2.1 Identify, and if possible, eliminate the cause

Pre-renal failure

Urine characteristics. Normal sediment, urine osmolality >700, urine sodium <10 mmol/l.
Causes. Dehydration, inadequate cardiac output.

Blood urea can also rise rapidly in a hypercatabolic patient with normal or slightly impaired renal function.

Intrinsic renal failure

Urine characteristics. Sediment contains tubular cells, cell and granular casts. Urine osmolality is osmolar with plasma, urine sodium >20 mmol/l.

Causes. Acute tubular necrosis (ATN), septicaemia, prolonged hypovolaemic hypotension, prolonged dehydration, nephrotoxic drugs (may be antibiotics in hospital practice), hyperbilirubinaemia, haemoglobin—mismatched blood transfusion or crush syndrome.

Other causes of intrinsic renal failure include glomerulonephritis, interstitial nephritis, pyelonephritis, and renal artery occlusion. These are rarely encountered as an acute situation and are strictly within the province of the nephrologist.

Post-renal failure
Obstruction of the renal outflow tract. Blockage of a urinary catheter is a common, and easily remediable, cause.

8.2.2 Treatment

Pre-renal failure
In the management of pre-renal failure, from whatever cause, the early insertion of a Swan–Ganz catheter for measurement of pulmonary artery wedge pressure (PAWP) is an invaluable guide to left ventricular function, and may also be used to determine cardiac output by thermodilution. A central venous catheter must be inserted, as well as an arterial line if facilities are available.

Dehydration. Correct by replacement of fluid with normal saline initially. If available, colloid should be replaced in the form of plasma protein fraction (PPF), or blood until central venous pressure, arterial pressure and PAWP are normal. If oliguria persists, intrinsic renal failure must be considered.

Renal blood flow. Renal blood flow and urine output may be improved by a dopamine infusion maintained at 3–4 µg/kg/min.

Cardiac output and blood pressure. If blood pressure and cardiac output remain low despite adequate fluid replacement as measured by CVP and PCWP, an inotrope should be started. Dopamine should be maintained at 3–4 µg/kg/min and initially dobutamine should be infused, followed by adrenaline or noradrenaline by infusion if dobutamine proves inadequate. If these drugs become necessary urgent transfer to an intensive therapy unit is mandatory.

Oliguria may follow acute regurgitation of the aortic or mitral valve. This requires urgent consideration of emergency valve replacement if established renal failure is to be avoided.

Intrinsic acute renal failure

Fluid balance. Insensible losses should be replaced with 500 ml (20 ml/h) of crystalloid as normal saline or dextrose saline. This may have to be increased if the patient has a high temperature or is in a hot environment.

Replace other fluid losses from nasogastric tube, abdominal or chest drains. Replace the urine output hourly with a volume equal to the output of the previous hour.

The most useful index of fluid balance is accurate daily weighing of the patient.

Diuretics. Diuresis may follow an infusion of mannitol 20 g intravenously. If there is a normal CVP, this may be repeated once if there is no response.

The use of diuretics is debatable; in the opinion of some nephrologists, a single dose of frusemide 500 mg infused in 100 ml of normal saline over 1 hour is worth trying in acute oliguria, provided that the patient is properly hydrated with a normal blood pressure and is not completely anuric. An alternative is to start a frusemide infusion at 60 mg/h for 8 hours initially. The dose can be progressively decreased after this once a diuresis has been established.

Other nephrologists believe that frusemide is rarely effective in established intrinsic acute renal failure and the use of such a large dose of frusemide may predispose to further renal damage or ototoxicity, particularly if the patient has high gentamicin levels as is often the case.

Vasodilatation. Improvement in renal blood flow may follow general vasodilatation if the patient is vasoconstricted. This policy should be approached with caution as the possible fall in blood pressure may be difficult to reverse. If this is attempted, a short-term acting drug like phentolamine is the most suitable.

Electrolyte balance. Potassium must be measured frequently in the early stages of treatment. Plasma potassium can be controlled temporarily with: Calcium resonium 15 g 6 hourly orally or 30 g 12

8

hourly rectally, dextrose 25 g and insulin 10 units intravenously. Correction of acidosis is by intravenous sodium bicarbonate.

Other electrolytes, urea and creatinine should be measured daily and adjustments made to electrolyte intake according to the electrolyte content of fluid losses.

Nutrition. If the patient is not catabolic, a protein intake of 50 g/day with 2000–3000 calories (8400–12600 joules) may suffice. More commonly hypercatabolism will increase both protein and calorie requirements to much higher levels. A formula for estimation of nitrogen loss can be found in the section on nutrition (see Section 10) and in the hypercatabolic patient replacement of nitrogen and calories should be based on this if possible. In practice, fluid restrictions make this very difficult in most cases of renal failure in the intensive therapy unit.

   If the patient is unable to eat, feeding should be by nasogastric route if possible. If not, intravenous feeding should be started as soon as possible. Calories can be provided from 50% glucose or fat; the choice of nitrogen source depends on how much is required.

Infection. Patients in renal failure are particularly susceptible to infection. Great care should be taken during the early stages in the handling of intravenous cannulae and central venous lines. A bladder catheter should only be used if it is really necessary.

Drugs. Many drugs, particularly antibiotics, must be given in reduced doses in renal failure. A detailed guide to drug dosage in renal failure can be found in: *British National Formulary,* The British Medical Association and The Pharmaceutical Society, London.

Dialysis. Dialysis and/or continuous haemofiltration should be considered if:
Blood urea is 40 mmol/l
Potassium is 6 mmol/l
There is evidence of fluid overload
There are uraemic symptoms, in particular, seizures, impending
   coma or vomiting
Uncontrollable metabolic acidosis develops

Summary

Fifty per cent of patients who develop acute renal failure die even if there is no other associated problem. In practice the presence of other disease processes and multi-organ failure increases this mortality considerably, even in experienced hands.

Although acute renal failure can be treated by peritoneal dialysis, recent developments with haemofiltration have meant that treatment is well within the scope of intensive therapy units without the need for a specialist nephrology unit. Despite this there is no doubt that if the clinical picture becomes complicated by multi-system failure, early transfer to a nephrology unit may increase the chances of survival.

8

Section 9
Diabetic Control

9

9.1 Hyperglycaemia, with or without acidosis

Incidence (district general hospital catchment area 200 000)
Twenty to thirty cases per annum

Mortality
Good centres 10–15%
Average district general hospital 20–25%
Geriatric patients 50%

Causes of death
1 Delay in diagnosis in primary or secondary health care.
2 Delay in treatment.
3 Failure to recognize coincidental or precipitating factors (e.g. infection, myocardial infarction, CVA).
4 Inadequate treatment of the diabetes:
  a not enough fluid
  b not enough insulin
  c not enough potassium
  d failure to correct acidosis
5 Inappropriate treatment; e.g. too much bicarbonate solution.
6 No nasogastric tube—aspiration pneumonia.

Priorities
1 Confirm diagnosis at bedside (accident and emergency or high care unit):
  a blood glucose (Glucostix (Ames) with or without a meter, or glycaeme B. M. sticks (Boehringer))
  b urinary ketones (ketostix, Ames)
2 Send blood to the laboratory. Tests for:
Blood glucose
Electrolytes and urea
Full blood picture (for PCV)
pH (and if possible bicarbonate/P_{O_2}/P_{CO_2}), blood ketones, blood for culture

9

9.1.1 Fluid balance

1 Set up i.v. infusion with or without central venous line.
2 Start infusion of normal saline ($Na^+ = 155$ mmol/l).
3 Rate of infusion:

1st hour	2 litres
2nd hour	1 litre
3rd hour, etc.	1 litre

Continue this rate of infusion until the patient is clinically rehydrated or the central venous pressure is normal.

Note: If plasma sodium rises to 155 mmol/l or more then hypotonic saline should be given. When blood glucose falls to 10 mmol/l or less, 5% or 10% dextrose should be given.

9.1.2 Insulin requirements

Start in accident and emergency or high care unit.
Intramuscular regimen (Alberti).

Note: Adequate hydration is essential otherwise insulin will not be absorbed. The following regimen is most useful if a high standard of nursing care is not available:

Regimen
1 At time zero, 20 units of intramuscular insulin (soluble, regular or Actrapid).
2 Then every hour, 6 units i.m. until the blood glucose falls to 10–15 mmol/l.
3 Then every 2 hours, 5 units i.m. until the blood glucose stabilizes at around 10 mmol/l. A three times daily insulin regimen may then be instituted when the patient starts to feed normally.

Intravenous regimen (Sonksen)
Infusions of insulin i.v. may be given using an infusion pump or by putting the insulin into an infusion of normal saline or dextrose.
   Rate of infusion 4 units per hour until the blood glucose is approximately 10 mmol/l then 1–0.5 units per hour to maintain the blood glucose of 7–10 mmol/l

9.1.3 Potassium requirements

A failure to correct potassium deficiency is a frequent cause of
death in diabetic ketoacidosis.

Replacement regimen

Plasma K$^+$ mmol/l	Dose of KCl: mmol/h i.v.
Greater than 5	0
4–5	13
Less than 4	26
Less than 3	39

9.1.4 Correction of acidosis

1 Only give bicarbonate solutions if pH is 7.1 or less.
2 Give 8.4% sodium bicarbonate solutions in *50 mmol (50 ml)
aliquots with 13 mmol of potassium added* to each aliquot. This
solution should be run in slowly over 20 minutes and after a 10
minute equilibration period the pH should be reassessed. If the pH
is 7.1 or less, step **2** should be repeated.

9.1.5 Other considerations

1 Chest X-ray.
2 ECG.
3 MSU for microscopy and culture.
4 Throat swabs.
5 Antibiotics.
6 Heparinization to prevent DVT and DIC in severely dehydrated
unconscious patients.
7 If patient remains oliguric/anuric after rehydration, with a normal
central venous pressure and a blood pressure of greater than
100 mmHg, treat with i.v. frusemide 120 mg. If this fails to produce
a diuresis, treat as acute renal failure.
8 Persistent hypotension (BP less than 80 mmHg) after 2 hours of
adequate hydration with a normal central venous pressure, give
blood (2 units).
9 If P_{O_2} less than 11 kPa (80 mmHg) give oxygen therapy.

9

Practical points

1 Blood glucose measured by bedside (Glucostix (Ames) or BM 20–800 strips (Boehringer)) initially every 30 minutes and then every 2 hours. Laboratory estimation of glucose, potassium, and pH every 2–4 hours.

2 Never leave blood glucose estimations to an inexperienced nurse. Inaccurate information is more dangerous than no information.

3 In the intravenous regimen Sonksen recommends the addition of albumin, polygeline, purified protein derivative or 2 ml of the patient's blood (to prevent adhesion of insulin to plastic surfaces).

4 If the intramuscular regimen fails, switch to intravenous regimen (common cause for failure is inadequate rehydration).

5 In the intravenous regimen if blood glucose does not fall, double intravenous dose. Common cause for failure of intravenous regimen is disconnection of the i.v. infusion or pump or inadvertent switching off of pump.

6 Plasma potassium may be high at presentation (i.e. greater than 5) because of intracellular acidosis. However, there may be a dramatic fall in the first hour and this must be expected and monitored. The ECG may be helpful but ST flattening and T wave inversion may not be seen until the plasma potassium is less than 2 mmol/l and this is too late!

7 If bicarbonate is given, an extra 13 mmol of potassium chloride must be given for every 50 mmol of bicarbonate.

8 Gastric atony-dilatation causes:
  a fluid and electrolyte imbalance
  b danger of aspiration pneumonia
Therefore *use an NG tube.*

9 As little as 50 mmol bicarbonate will relieve distressing hyperventilation due to acidosis

10 For every mmol of bicarbonate given, a mmol of sodium is given. There is therefore a danger of hypernatraemia, consequent hyperosmolarity of plasma and therefore intracellular dehydration which might lead to death.

9.2 Surgery in diabetes

9.2.1 Cold surgery

Insulin-treated diabetics
1 Admit 3 days pre-op. and stabilize on a thrice daily insulin regimen (Actrapid/soluble/regular insulin with a small dose of Monotard/NPH to cover the overnight period). Aim for blood glucose 3–7 mmol/l.
2 One day pre-op. change to short-acting insulin only (e.g. Actrapid thrice daily).

Suggested PIG regimen
On day of operation set up i.v. infusion ('PIG regimen') of:
Potassium as KCL 1 g (13 mmol)
Insulin Actrapid/soluble/regular insulin 10 units
Glucose as 10% Dextrose in 500 ml
This 500 ml solution to be run in 4–5 hourly until oral feeding restarts. The insulin dose should be varied as follows:

Blood sugar	Insulin dose
Up to 5 mmol/l	5 units
5–9 mmol/l	10–15 units
10–19 mmol/l	15–20 units
Greater than 20 mmol/l	20–25 units/500 ml

The blood glucose, urea and electrolytes should be checked before operation and 2–3 hours after starting infusion. Thereafter the blood sugar should be checked 4 hourly and the urea and electrolytes 8 hourly. Potassium inclusion in the regimen should be varied according to the serum potassium.
When oral feeding begins the infusion should be stopped and the patient should be restabilized on a thrice daily Actrapid regimen with the three main meals.

Other considerations
1 If there is evidence of infection, the pre-operative dose will be increased by 20% or more.

2 If steroids are administered, the pre-operative dose will also be increased by 20% or more.

3 If the patient is fed intravenously, it is important to maintain normoglycaemia (to aid healing and reduce infection) by using an insulin infusion. This is best done with a separate line and an infusion pump.

4 When using the PIG or any other infusion regimen it is essential to have a separate i.v. line from that which is being used for other infusions such as blood and saline.

Non-insulin-treated diabetics

If diabetic control is poor, it is better to admit and stabilize on insulin and then use the PIG regimen as above.

If control is good (blood glucose 2 hours after a meal 3–7 mmol/l), then on the day of operation the patient should receive no food and no oral hypoglycaemic agent. Long-acting oral hypoglycaemic agent such as chloropropamide or glibenclamide should be stopped 24 hours pre-operatively. Blood glucose should be monitored pre-operatively and during the operation using Dextrostix (Ames) or Glycaemie BM strips (Boehringer). If the blood glucose falls below 3 mmol/l then i.v. 5% dextrose should be given to maintain a blood glucose of 3–7 mmol/l.

After minor procedures the patient should be restarted on diet with or without a sulphonylurea with the first normal meal. However, in major procedures it may be necessary to give the patient insulin to maintain the blood glucose at 3–7 mmol/l, as above.

Section 10
Fluids, Electrolytes and Nutrition

10.1 Body compartment volumes of the neonate, child and adult

	Neonate	Child	Adult
Total body water	75–80% wt	60–65% wt	50–60% wt
Blood volume (ml/kg)	82–87	75–80	55–70
Plasma volume (ml/kg)	50–55	45–50	35–45
ECF	45–50% wt	30–35% wt	20–25% wt
Cardiac output	900 ml/min	3 l/min	5 l/min
O_2 consumption	7 ml/kg/min	5 ml/kg/min	3.5 ml/kg/min
Blood pressure (systolic)	45–75 mmHg	80–100 mmHg	120–150 mmHg

10.2 Electrolyte contents of body fluids

Fluid	Na^+ (mmol/l)	K^+ (mmol/l)	HCO_3^- (mmol/l)	Cl^- (mmol/l)	H_2O (ml/24 h)	pH
Sweat	50	10		45	500–1000	
Gastric	60	15	0.15	140	2500	1.5–3
Saliva	112	20	10–20	30	500–1500	5–6.5
Bile	140	6	30–50	90	300–1000	5.7–8.6
Pancreatic	130	6	100	60	300–1500	7.7–8
Small gut	120	8	20–40	100	1000–3000	6–7
Diarrhoea	75	30	20–80		500+	
Stools	30	60	20–60	40	100	6.5–8
Urine	70	40		80	1000–2000	5.5–7
CSF	140	4	25	130	100–160	7.32–7.40

10

10.3 Electrolyte bottle contents per litre

Bottle	Strength (%)	pH	Osmolality	Na$^+$	Ions K$^+$	(mmol/l) Cl$^-$	HCO$_3^-$	CHO (g/l)	Protein (g/l)	Cal	Misc. (mmol)
NaCl (normal)	0.9	5	308	150	0	150	0	0	0	0	
NaCl ($\frac{1}{2}$ normal)	0.45	5.2	154	77	0	77	0	0	0	0	
NaCl ($\frac{1}{3}$ normal)	0.30	5.5	114	51	0	51	0	0	0	0	
Dextrose saline dextrose / $\frac{1}{5}$ isotonic saline	4 / 0.18	4.5	300	30	0	30	0	40	0	150	
Dextrose saline $\frac{1}{2}$ strength dextrose / $\frac{1}{2}$ isotonic saline	5 / 0.45	4.5	300	77	0	77	0	50	0	188	
Dextrose 5%	5	4	278	0	0	0	0	50	0	188	
Dextrose 10%	10		523	0	0	0	0	100	0	375	
Ringer lactate (Hartmann's)		6.5	280	131	5	112	29 (as lact.)	0	0	9	9 {Mg^{++} 1, Ca^{++} 1}
Ringer lactate $\frac{1}{2}$ strength in 4.5% dextrose		6	280	65	2.5	56	14 (as lact.)	45	0	180	

Dextran 40 in 5% dextrose				0		0		50	0	205	
Dextran 40 in isotonic saline				144		144		0	0	0	
Dextran 70 in isotonic saline				144		144		0	0	0	
Dextran 70 in 5% dextrose				0		0		50	0	205	
NaHCO₃	8.4	8	2008	1000		0	1000		0	0	
NaHCO₃	4.2	7.5	1004	500		0	500		0	0	
NaHCO₃	1.4		484	167		0	167		0	0	
Mannitol	10		550								
Mannitol	20		1100								
Ammonium chloride	$\frac{1}{6}$ M		338	0		168	0		0	0	NH_4^+ 168
Na lactate	$\frac{1}{6}$ M			167		0	167 (as lact.)		0	0	
Blood/l	3.5	<6		140	15+	103					
Haemaccel				145	5	145				160	Ca^{++} 6.25
Hespan	6%			150		150			0	0	
Human plasma protein/l				150	2	120			39		
Gelofusine	4			154	0.4	125			45	184	Ca^{++} 0.4 / Mg 0.4
Packed cell/l				10	30+	26					
Plasma/l			290	152	15+	100					Ca^{++} 2.5

10

10.4 Infusion nomogram

Drip rates for different infusion sets. Place a ruler across the chart at the drops/ml drop size and the amount of fluid needed per day. Read off the drops per minute.

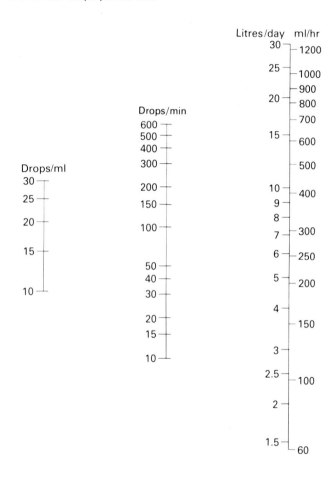

10.5 Paediatric fluid and electrolyte requirements

10.5.1 Fluid requirement in children (Liverpool) method

First 10 kg body weight—100 ml/kg/day = 4 ml/kg/h
Next 10 kg body weight—50 ml/kg/day = 2 ml/kg/h
Additional body weight—20 ml/kg/day = 0.8 ml/kg/h

For example, a child of 30 kg needs 1000 + 500 + 200 ml/day. Less fit children post-op. need less, i.e.
70–80 ml/kg/day for first 10 kg body weight
30–40 ml/kg/day for next 10 kg body weight

10

10.5.2 A paediatric guide

The chart below shows average healthy values ±15%, so will only give a guide to parameters.

	Age (years)													
	0	0.25	0.5	0.75	1	2	3	4	5	6	7	8	9	10
Weight (kg)	3.5	5	7	8.5	10	13	15	17	19	21	23	25	28	32
Height (cm)	50	60	65	70	75	86	97	104	110	115	123	131	135	140
Blood volume (litre)	0.2	0.4	0.52	0.65	0.75	0.9	1.05	1.22	1.37	1.52	1.7	1.9	2.06	2.4
Haemoglobin (g)	18	10	11	11.5	12	12.7	13.1	13.3	13.5	13.6	13.7	13.8	13.9	14
Haematocrit (%)	61	30	32	34	36	37	37.6	38.2	38.8	39.5	40	40.5	41	42
Water (ml/kg/day)	130	125	120	115	110	102	95	93	90	86	82	78	76	75
Na and K (mmol/kg/day)	4	3.7	3.3	3	2.8	2.5	2	1.98	1.95	1.90	1.85	1.8	1.75	1.7
Calories (kcal/day)	112	111	109	107	105	101	98	97	96	93	90	85	80	75
Urine (ml/day)	280	300	340	370	400	450	500	530	560	640	700	750	800	850
Insensible loss (ml/kg)	31	30	29	28	27.5	27	26.5	26	25	24	23	22	21	20

10.6 Electrolyte and nutritional requirements per kg

	Adult	Child >10 kg	Deficiency
Energy/kg	30 kcal (125 kJ)	75 kcal (450 kJ)	
Nitrogen	160 mg	300 mg	
Protein	1 g	1.75 g	
Water	30–35 ml	100 ml	
Glucose	2–3 g	15 g	
Fat	2 g	4 g	
Sodium	1–2 mmol	3 mmol	
Potassium	1 mmol	3 mmol	
Chloride	1–2 mmol	2–3 mmol	
Calcium	0.19 mmol	0.75 mmol	
Phosphorus	0.25 mmol	0.3 mmol	Fits
Iron	1.05 µmol	1.4 µmol	Microcytic anaemia
Magnesium	0.25 mmol	0.6 mmol	
Zinc	2.3 µmol	12.5 µmol	Eczema, bad healing
Manganese	0.6 µmol	1 µmol	
Copper	0.9 µmol	3 µmol	Leucopenia
Chromium	0.01 µmol		
Fluoride	0.75 µmol	3 µmol	
Iodine	0.05 µmol	1.5 µmol	Hypothyroid
Selenium	5.7 nmol		
Molybdenum	3 nmol		
Thiamin (B1)	0.04 mg	0.06 mg	
Riboflavin (B2)	0.05 mg	0.08 mg	Stomatitis
Niacin	0.6 mg	0.8 mg	Dermatitis
Pyridoxine (B6)	0.06 mg	0.1 mg	Anaemia
Folate	6 µg	100 µg	Megaloblastic anaemia
Vitamin B12	0.07 µg	0.2 µg	Megaloblastic anaemia
Pantothenic acid	0.2 mg		
Biotin	1.86 µg		Dermatitis
Vitamin A	14.2 µg	30 µg	
Vitamin C	1.4 mg	2 mg	
Vitamin D	0.07 µg	10 µg	Osteomalacia
Vitamin K	1 µg	1.5 µg	PTT reduced
Vitamin E	0.15 mg	0.5 mg	

10

10.7 Basal metabolic rate

The following chart shows basal metabolic rates in energy/m^2 body surface/h.

Age (years)	Males kcal	Males mJ	Females kcal	Females mJ
3	51.1–68.8	0.215–0.288	46.4–62.6	0.194–0.261
5	47.7–65	0.198–0.271	44.9–61.1	0.288–0.255
7	43.4–60.7	0.181–0.253	42.1–58.3	0.176–0.243
9	39.6–56.3	0.165–0.235	38.2–54.5	0.159–0.227
11	37.7–52.2	0.157–0.218	35.1–50.6	0.146–0.211
13	36–49.3	0.150–0.206	33.2–45.1	0.139–0.188
16	33.7–46.9	0.141–0.196	31.3–40.8	0.131–0.171
19	32.7–45	0.137–0.188	29.7–39.3	0.124–0.164
22	32.4–43.1	0.135–0.180	29.2–38.8	0.122–0.162
30	31.4–41.4	0.131–0.173	29.2–38.9	0.122–0.163
40	30.5–40.5	0.127–0.169	27.8–37.5	0.116–0.157
50	28.8–38.8	0.120–0.162	27.1–36.7	0.113–0.153
60	28.1–38.1	0.117–0.159	26.5–36.1	0.111–0.151
70	27.4–37.4	0.114–0.156	25.9–35.5	0.108–0.148

10.8 Parenteral nutrition

10.8.1 Total parenteral nutrition (TPN) bottle contents per litre

Bottle	Strength	pH	Osmol	Na	K	Cl	N_2	CHO	Prot.	kcal	Mg	Misc. adds (mmol)
Sugar solutions												
Dextrose	10	5.6	523	0	0	0	0	100	0	400	0	0
Dextrose	20	5.6	1250	0	0	0	0	200	0	800	0	0
Dextrose	50	5.6	3800	0	0	0	0	500	0	2000	0	0
Ethanol	5		1500	0	0	0	0	50	0	350	0	0
Fructose	25		1500	0	0	0	0	250	0	1000	0	0
Glucoplex	1000		1500	50	30	67	0	240	0	1000	2.5	PO_4 18:Zn 0.046
Glucoplex	1600		2800	50	30	67	0	400	0	1600	2.5	PO_4 18:Zn 0.046
Glucoven	1000		1500	50	30	67	0	240	0	1000	2.5	PO_4 18:Zn 0.046
Glucoven	1600		2800	50	30	67	0	400	0	1600	2.5	PO_4 18:Zn 0.046
Laevuflex	20	5.5	1250	0	0	0	0	200	0	810	0	Fructose
Normodex	15	5.2	945	40	20	40	0	150	0	615	1.5	Lactate 23
Sorbitol	30	6	2100	0	0	0	0	300	0	1200	0	0
Amino acid solutions												
Aminofusin	600	6.8		40	30	14	7.6	100	48	626	5	+Sorbitol
Aminofusin	1000	6.8		40	30	14	7.6	250	48	1000	5	+Sorbitol+ethanol
Aminofusin	Forte			40	30	28	15.2	0	95	405	5	
Aminoplasmal	L3			48	25	18	4.8	0	30	121	2.5	PO_4 9
Aminoplasmal	L5			48	25	31	8	0	50	202	2.5	PO_4 9
Aminoplasmal	L10			48	25	62	16.1	0	100	404	2.5	PO_4 9

10

Bottle	Strength	pH	Osmol	Na	K	Cl	N_2	CHO	Prot.	kcal	Mg	Misc. adds (mmol)
Aminoplasmal	Ped			50	25	15	7.4	0	46	202	2.5	
Aminoplex	5	7.4	350	35	28	43	6	175	35	1000	4.5	+Sorbitol+ethanol
Aminoplex	12	7.4	800	35	30	67	12.4	0	78	316	2.5	
Aminoplex	14	7.4	960	35	30	81	13.4	0	84	340	0	
Aminoplex	24	7.4		35	30	67	25	0	156	620	2.5	
Aminoven	12			35	30	67	12.4	0	78	310	2.5	
Freamine	8.5			10	0	2	13	0	81	333	0	PO_4 10
Freamine	10	6.5		10	0	2	15.3	0	96	393	0	PO_4 10
Nephramine				5	0	2	6.5	0	41	200	0	Essent. amino acids
Perifusin	5			40	30	9	5	0	31	132	5	
Plasmalyte	148			140	5	98	0	0	0	19	1.5	Gluconate 23
Plasmalyte	148			140	5	98	0	50	0	210	1.5	Gluconate 23
Plasmalyte	M			40	16	40	0	50	0	200	1.5	Ca 2.5: lactate 12
Synthamin	9	6		73	60	70	9.3	0	57	236	5	PO_4 30
Synthamin	14	6		73	60	70	14.3	0	90	363	5	PO_4 30
Synthamin	17	6		73	60	70	16.9	0	105	429	5	PO_4 30
Vamin N	9	5.5		50	20	55	9.4	0	60	239	1.5	Ca 2.5
Vamin glucose		5.2	1275	50	20	55	9.4	0	60	650	1.5	Ca 2.5
Vamin	14			100	50	100	13.5	100	84	333	8	Ca 5:SO_4 8
Intralipid	10	7	280	0	0	0	0	0	0	1000	0	Soya 100 g:PO_4 15
Intralipid	20	7	330	0	0	0	0	0	0	2000	0	Soya 200 g:PO_4 15
Travamulsion	10	7	280	0	0	0	0	0	0	1000	0	Soya 100 g
Travamulsion	20	7	330	0	0	0	0	0	0	2000	0	Soya 200 g

10.8.2 Calorific values of nutrients

	Calorific value (cal/g)	Respiratory quotient (RQ)
Fat	9	0.7
Alcohol	7	0.66
Protein	4.2	0.8
CHO	4	1

RQ normally 0.8 (on average diet).

10.8.3 Factors to be considered when using parenteral nutrition

Assessment of nutritional requirements
Assessment from loss of body weight:

10% loss over predicted weight from height and age = mild
   malnutrition

20% loss over predicted weight from height and age = moderate
   malnutrition

30% loss over predicted weight from height and age = severe
   malnutrition

Assessment from anthropometric measurements:

Skinfold thickness over triceps, biceps, scapula, or supra-iliac
   crests.

Mid-arm circumference. Arm muscle circumference = arm
   circumference − 3 times triceps thickness.

   There are numerous nomograms for estimating requirements of
TPN from these data. Respiratory function tests, oxygen
consumption, anaemia and plasma proteins will also demonstrate
the degree and progress in TPN.

10

Assessments of nitrogen loss:

1 Urine nitrogen loss (g/24 h) = urine urea (mmol/l) × 24 h urine
volume (l) × 0.0336.

2 Non urine nitrogen loss $(g/24\ h)$ = change in blood urea over 24 h (mmol/l) $\times$ wt (kg) $\times$ 0.0168.
3 Proteinuria nitrogen loss $(g/24\ h)$ = proteinuria $(g/24\ h)$ $\times$ 0.16.
4 Skin/faeces loss in 24 h = 1 g (approx.).

Total 24 h loss = **1** + **2** + **3** + **4** $(g\ N_2)$.
1 g nitrogen = 6.25 g protein = 25.3 g wet muscle.

Remember that normal losses of 1 g N_2/kg/day increase by:
15% in post-operative patients
25% in long bone fractures
50% in severe infections
100% in severe burns

In planning ideal TPN give:
1 Glucose as the carbohydrate
2 Fats as soya fat in equicaloric levels
3 Nitrogen as amino acids but only little glycine
4 Insulin to help carbohydrate and amino acid metabolism. Aim for blood sugar of 7–10 mmol/l, by giving 4–6 units/h. Give 2–3 units/h if blood sugar below 4. Give 9 units/h if blood sugar above 12 mmol/l
5 150:1 calories to grams of nitrogen
Add trace elements, Mg PO_4, electrolytes, vitamin K and other fat- and water-soluble vitamins.

To correct an apparently low calcium:
Corrected calcium (mmol/l) = measured calcium (mmol/l) + 40 − serum albumin (g/l)

Remember that:
1 Ideally enteral feeding is safe and efficient and should be used whenever possible. Use cyclical boluses or continuous feeding. Only use TPN in cases of *gut* failure, or very sick patients.
2 Carnitine is essential to help fat metabolism and is made in the liver by amino acids.
3 Phosphate deficiency occurs below 0.35 mmol/l in blood. This leads to anorexia, weakness, tremor, confusion, fits and coma.
4 Magnesium deficiency causes fasciculation, tetany, vertigo and depression.

5 Zinc deficiency occurs after urinary losses of 50–100 µmol/day. This leads to skin rashes, hair loss, diarrhoea, poor wound healing and depression.

6 Copper deficiency occurs with urinary losses of 5 mmol/day. This leads to hypochromic anaemia, neutropaenia and osteoporosis.

7 Folate deficiency occurs after a short period of malnutrition, and causes pancytopaenia.

10.8.4 Suggested 3 litre bag premixed feed

Plain		Intralipid	
Vamin glucose 10%	1500 ml	Vamin glucose 10%	1500 ml
Dextrose 50%	1000 ml	Dextrose 20%	1000 ml
Dextrose 20%	500 ml	Intralipid 20%	500 ml
Folic acid	6–10 mg	Folic acid	10 mg
Potassium	100 mmol	Potassium	92 mmol
Sodium	90 mmol	Sodium	98 mmol
Phosphate	60 mmol	Phosphate	38 mmol
Solvito	1 vial	Solvito	1 vial
Addamel	1 vial	Addamel	1 vial
Insulin	80–120 units	Vitalipid	1 vial

10

10.8.5 Enteral feed per 1000 ml

Name	kcal	cal/N	Prot	Fat	CHO	Na	K	Cl	Ca	P	Mg	Mn	Cu	Zn	Osmol	Type
Clinifeed:																
Favour	1000	145/1	38	33	140	30	28	32	12	11	8	36	15	120	335	Normal
Iso	1000	200/1	28	41	130	15	38	29	15	14	5	4	15	135	270	Normal
Protein Rich	1000	79/1	60	22	140	25	43	26	6	18	4	54	8	112	399	Normal
Elemental 028	800	225/1	20	13	156	22	24	19	9	13	5	22	12	125	720	Elemental
Enrich	1040	148/1	38	35	153	35	38	38	17	22	11	54	21	225	400	Normal
Ensure	1000	153/1	35	35	137	35	38	38	12	16	8	45	15	169	380	Normal
Ensure Plus	1500	125/1	62	50	200	51	47	45	27	34	17	95	31	360	500	Normal
Flexical	1000	253/1	22	34	152	15	32	28	14	16	8	45	15	150	550	Peptide
Fortison:																
Plus	1500	167/1	50	65	179	35	38	22	12	16	6	70	15	105	320	Normal
Standard	1000	131/1	40	40	120	35	38	22	12	16	6	70	15	105	260	Normal
Fresubin	1000	140/1	38	34	138	33	32	33	19	19	7	27	15	112	300	Normal
Isocal	980	174/1	32	42	126	21	32	28	15	16	8	55	16	153	300	Normal
Liquisorb	1000	130/1	40	40	118	45	45	50	16	17	8	22	19	90	270	Normal
Nutauxil	1000	140/1	38	34	138	33	32	33	12	19	5	27	15	112	350	Normal
Osmolite	1000	126/1	42	35	134	38	38	38	18	23	12	64	21	243	263	Normal
Nutranel	1000	130/1	40	10	187	20	35	24	11	12	4	72	15	105	410	Peptide
Peptisorbon	1000	126/1	45	13	175	60	30	40	12	19	8	27	15	112	400	Peptide
Reabilan	1000	175/1	31	39	131	27	28	52	11	14	9	27	19	124	300	Peptide
Trisorbon	1000	129/1	40	40	119	42	42	53	13	19	7	22	15	112	215	Normal
Vivonex	1000	280/1	18	2	207	37	30	51	13	18	9	28	17	125	550	Elemental

Section 11
Pharmacology

11

11.1 General drugs

11.1.1 Introduction—Pharmacology: drugs and doses

The drugs detailed in this section are some of those used most often in hospital practice. Antibiotics and those drugs peculiar to anaesthesia are not included here but are to be found in Section 11.2, p. 188–192 and Sections 2.4 and 2.5, pp. 11–27, respectively.

There are three columns in the general drug list table:

1 The non-proprietary name of the drug. A list of proprietary names and their non-proprietary equivalents are to be found in Section 11.3, pp. 193–212.

2 The usual dose for an average-sized adult, including frequency of administration and possible routes. In many cases the initial dose of a drug is increased after a short period to evaluate the clinical effect and these are indicated by the suffix 'initially'.

3 The paediatric dose. In some instances the drug is specifically not recommended for children and this is indicated. In others, there is no mention of a paediatric dose or it is clearly irrelevant, and these have been left blank. A general guide to dosage in paediatrics is given in the table below.

A comprehensive guide to prescribing both in general and in particular situations can be found in the *British National Formulary*, which is published by the British Medical Association and The Pharmaceutical Society of Great Britain and is frequently updated.

If any doubt exists about the dose of a drug, particularly in children, it is advisable to check with the manufacturer's data sheet, your pharmacy, or a paediatrician.

11

11.1.2 Solution strength conversion table

This is used for drugs and vapours, i.e. 1% solution contains 1 g of substance in 100 ml of solution.

Ratio	Percentage in solution	Concentration (mg/ml)
1:400 000	0.00025	0.0025
1:200 000	0.002	0.02
1:100 000	0.001	0.01
1:10 000	0.01	0.1
1:5 000	0.02	0.2
1:4 000	0.025	0.25
1:2 000	0.05	0.5
1:1 000	0.1	1
1:500	0.2	2
1:400	0.25	2.5
1:100	1	10

11.1.3 Paediatric prescribing regimen

Age	Average wt (kg)	Proportion of adult dose (%)
2 months	3.2	10
4 months	6.5	15
1 year	10	25
5 years	18	33
7 years	23	50
12 years	37	75
15 years	55	85
Adult	66	100

11.1.4 General drug list

Drug	Adult dose	Paediatric dose
Acebutolol	200 mg b.d. o initially 5–25 mg i.v. slowly	
Acetazolamide	250 mg 6 h o, i.m., i.v.	Infant: 125 mg/day Child: 125–750 mg/day DD o
Acetohexamide	0.25–1.5 g D o	
ACTH	See corticotrophin	
Adrenaline 1/1000 (Also see Section 6.5)	0.5 mg = 0.5 ml s.c. 1 mg in 100 ml = 10 µg/ml by i.v. infusion	
Alfacalcidol	1 µg D o	20 kg adult dose 20 kg 50 ng/kg D o
Allopurinol	100–200 mg/day o initially Then 200–600 mg/day o	10–20 mg/kg/day o
Amiloride	5–20 mg/day o	
Aminophylline (Also see Section 6.5)	100–300 mg o 360 mg b.d. rect. 250 mg i.v. slowly Infusion: 250 mg in 500 ml in 6 h	*Age*　*Oral*　*Rectal* 0–1 yr　10–25 mg　12.5–25 　　　　　　　　mg b.d. 1–5 yr　25–50 mg　50–100 　　　　　　　　mg b.d. 6–12 yr　50–100　100–200 　　　　mg　　mg b.d.
Amiodarone	200 mg tds o 5 mg/kg i.v. infusion over 30 min in 250 ml 5% dextrose Then up to 1.2 g in 24 h	
Amitryptiline	25 mg t.d.s. o initially 10–20 mg q.d.s. i.m., i.v.	Enuresis only
Amylobarbitone	200 mg o Up to 500 mg i.m. Up to 1 g i.v.	
Ancrod	Initial dose: 2–3 mg/kg in normal saline 50–500 ml in 8 h infusion Maintain: 2 units/kg in 25 ml i.v. bolus slowly 12 h Lab. control	
Aprotinin	500 000 KI units stat 200 000 KI units 4 h i.v. infusion	As adult in proportion to body wt
Aspirin	600 mg 4 h o 300 mg/day for anticoagulation	1–2 yr: 75–150 mg 6 h 3–5 yr: 225–300 mg 8 h 6–12 yr: 300–400 mg 6 h

11

Drug	Adult dose	Paediatric dose
Atenolol	50–100 mg daily o 2.5 mg i.v. slowly (max. 10 mg in 20 min) 0.15 mg/kg i.v. over 20 min 12 h	
Atropine	0.3–1 mg i.m. i.v. (See also Section 11.2)	0.02 mg/kg
Azathioprine	1–4 mg/kg/day o 1–2.5 mg/kg i.v. I slowly	As adult
Bendrofluazide	2.5–10 mg daily o	
Benztropine	1–2 mg/day o initially 1–2 mg i.v.	
Betamethasone	0.5–5 mg/day o 4–20 mg 6 h i.m., i.v.	1/4–1/2 adult dose o 0–1 yr: 1 mg i.v. 1–5 yr: 2 mg i.v. 6–12 yr: 3 mg i.v.
Bethanidine	10 mg t.d.s. o initially	
Bretylium	5 mg/kg i.m. Repeat 6–8 h	
Bumetanide	1 mg daily o 1–2 mg i.m., i.v. 2–5 mg by i.v. infusion.	
Buprenorphine	0.2–0.4 mg 6–8 h subling. 0.3–0.6 mg 6–8 h i.m.	Not in children
Calcium chloride	2.5–5 mmol i.v.	
Calcium gluconate	Calcium deficiency	See manufacturer's data sheet
Captopril	12.5 mg b.d. o initially	
Carbamazepine	100–200 mg b.d., t.d.s. o initially	10–20 mg/kg/day o DD
Carbenoxolone	100 mg t.d.s. o initially	
Carbimazole	10 mg t.d.s. o initially	>7 yr: 5 mg t.d.s. o
Chloral hydrate	1–2 g o	30–50 mg/kg o (max. 1 g)
Chlordiazepoxide	10 mg t.d.s. o (Higher dose possible) 50–100 mg i.m.	5–20 mg/day DD o
Chlormethiazole	Sedation: 1 capsule = 192 mg 2 capsules o *nocte* Higher dose in alcohol withdrawal Infusion i.v. 8 mg/ml, 1 ml/min *CAUTION: Overdose = anaesthesia*	
Chlormezanone	200 mg t.d.s. o 400 mg o *nocte*	Not in children
Chloroquine	(See manufacturer's data sheet)	
Chlorothiazide	500 mg–2 mg daily o	

Drug	Adult dose	Paediatric dose
Chlorpheniramine	4 mg t.d.s. o 10–20 mg s.c., i.m., i.v. (max. 40 mg/24 h)	Syrup: 4 mg in 10 ml 0–1 yr: 2.5 ml b.d. o 1–5 yr: 2.5–5 ml t.d.s. o
Chlorpromazine	25 mg t.d.s. o. initially 25–50 mg 6–8 h i.m. 5–10 mg i.v.	Under 5 yr: 5–10 mg o, i.m. Over 5 yr: $\frac{1}{3}$–$\frac{1}{2}$ adult dose t.d.s. o i.m.
Chlorpropamide	250–500 mg D o (100–125 mg in older patients)	
Chlorthalidone	50–100 mg D o	Up to 10 kg: 5 mg/kg *alt die* o Up to 5 yr: 50 mg *alt die* o Over 5 yr: 50–100 mg *alt die* o
Choline theophyllinate	100–400 mg q.d.s o	Syrup: 62.5 mg/5 ml 3–6 yr: 5–10 ml t.d.s. o Over 6 yr: 100 mg t.d.s. o (tab)
Chymotrypsin	20 mg b.d. o 3 days Maintain: 10 mg b.d. o	
Cimetidine	200 mg t.d.s., 400 mg *nocte* o 200 mg 4–6 h i.m., i.v.	20–40 mg/kg/day DD o, i.v.
Clobazam	10 mg t.d.s. o	Over 3 yr: $\frac{1}{2}$ adult dose
Clofibrate	Over 65 kg: 500 mg q.d.s. o Under 65 kg: 500 mg t.d.s. o	
Clomipramine	10 mg/day o initially 25 mg 6 times/day i.m. 25–50 mg i.v. infusion over 2 h	
Clonazepam	1 mg/day o initially 1 mg i.v.—Slow B. I	Initially: Infant: 0.25 mg/day o Child: 0.5 mg/day o 0.5 mg i.v. slowly
Clonidine	0.05–0.1 mg t.d.s. o initially 0.15–0.3 mg i.v. slowly	
Codeine phosphate	10–60 mg 4 h o 30 mg 4–6 h i.m.	3 mg/kg/day DD o
Corticotrophin (ACTH)	40 i.u. D s.c., i.m. initially Reduce dose to response	*See* manufacturer's data sheet
Cortisone acetate	Variable dose, usually 25–100 mg daily DD o, i.m., i.v.	
Cyanocobalamin	1 mg. 10 doses at 2 day intervals Then 1 mg/month i.m.	As adult initially then depends on response
Cyclandelate	400 mg t.d.s. o	Not in children
Cyclizine	50 mg t.d.s. o, i.m., i.v.	1–10 yr: 25 mg t.d.s. o Not by injection
Cyclopenthiazide	0.25–0.5 mg D o	

11

Drug	Adult dose	Paediatric dose
Dantrolene	25 mg daily o initially Hyperpyrexia: 1 mg/kg i.v. Repeat up to 10 mg/kg max.	
Debrisoquine	10–20 mg D. or b.d. o	Not in children
Desferrioxamine	Iron poisoning: 5–10 g in 50–100 ml water o 1–2 g 3–12 h i.m. Infusion i.v. 15 mg/kg/h max. 80 mg/kg/24 h	As in adult
Dexamethasone	0.5–2 g daily o 0.5–20 mg daily DD i.m., i.v. High doses, see manufacturer's data sheet	Reduce dose in proportion to weight
Dextromoramide	5 mg o, s.c., i.m. initially Increase to max. 20 mg/dose 10 mg rect	0.08 mg/kg but not recommended
Dextropropoxyphene	65 mg t.d.s., q.d.s o Usually used as compound preparation with paracetamol, e.g. Distalgesic tab. 2 6 h o	Not in children
Diamorphine	5 mg o, i.m., i.v. Extradural: 2–5 mg in 10 ml of normal saline.	
Diazepam	2.5–10 mg o, i.m., i.v.	0.1 mg/kg
Diazoxide	300 mg i.v. rapidly	5 mg/kg i.v.
Dichloralphenazone	2–3 650 mg tab, *nocte* o	Elixir: 225 mg in 5 ml Up to 1 yr: 2.5–5 ml 1–5 yr: 5–10 ml 6–12 yr: 10–20 ml
Diclofenac	75 mg b.d., o, i.m. Not i.v.	Not in children
Dicyclomine	10–20 mg t.d.s. o	Syrup: 10 mg in 5 ml Up to 6 months: 5 mg t.d.s. o 6 months–2 yr: 5–10 mg t.d.s. o. 2–12 yr: 10–20 mg t.d.s. o
Diflunisal	500 mg b.d. o	Not in children
Digoxin	0.25–0.5 mg D o, i.m. Load dose: 0.5–1 mg i.m., i.v. repeat after 4 h	0.01–0.02 mg/kg repeat in 6 h then daily. All routes
Dihydrocodeine	30 mg 4–6 h o 50 mg 4–6 h i.m.	Over 4 years 0.5–1 mg/kg 4–6 h o
Diltiazem	60 mg t.d.s. o initially	
Dimenhydrinate	50–100 mg t.d.s. o	1–6 yr: 12.5–25 mg t.d.s. o 6–12 yr: 25–50 mg t.d.s. o

Drug	Adult dose	Paediatric dose
Dimercaprol	2.5–3 mg/kg 4 h i.m. initially	
Diphenoxylate	1 dose 4 tab, then 2 tab 6 h o	1–3 yr: 1 tab b.d. 4–8 yr: 1 tab t.d.s. 9–12 yr: 1 tab q.d.s. 13–16 yr: 2 tab t.d.s.
Dipipanone + cyclizine	1 tab 6 h o	Not in children
Dipyridamole	100–200 mg t.d.s. o	5 mg/kg/day DD
Disopyramide	100 mg 6 h o 2 mg/kg i.v. slowly. Max. 150 mg Infusion: 0.4 mg/kg/h Max. 800 mg/24 h	
Distigmine	5 mg daily o. Increases to max. 20 mg/day 0.5 mg i.m.	Up to 10 mg daily o, depending on age
Dobutamine (Also see Section 6.5)	Infusion: 50 mg in 100 ml; rate depends on effect	
Dopamine (Also see Section 6.5)	Infusion: 200 mg in 100 ml; rate depends on effect: usually 5–10 µg/kg/min	
Doxapram	Infusion: 2 mg/ml 0.5–4 mg/min	
Enalapril	2.5–5 mg D o initially Max. 40 mg D	
Edrophonium	2 mg i.v. initially. 1 mg increments up to 10 mg	Up to 35 kg: 1 mg i.v. 2 mg i.m. Over 35 kg: 2 mg i.v., 5 mg i.m.
Ephedrine	15–60 mg t.d.s. o Up to 10 mg i.v. 10–30 mg i.m.	Up to 1 yr: 7.5 mg t.d.s. o 1–5 yr: 15 mg t.d.s. o 6–12 yr: 30 mg t.d.s. o
Ergometrine	0.5–1 mg o 0.25–0.5 mg i.m., i.v.	
Ergotamine	1–2 mg o. Repeat $\frac{1}{2}$ hourly up to total of 6 mg/migraine attack 1 mg i.v., i.m.	
Ethacrynic acid	50 mg D o i.v. initially	Over 2 yr: 25 mg daily o Not parenteral
Ethamivan	50–100 mg i.v. up to max. 250 mg	Oral solution: 12 drops = 25 mg Lingual absn. Infant: 6 drops Child: 12 drops

11

Drug	Adult dose	Paediatric dose
Ethamsylate	500 mg q.d.s. o, i.m., i.v. 1 g i.m., i.v. stat	Infant: 12.5 mg/kg 6 h i.m., i.v. Child: 250 mg 6 h o, i.v. 500–750 mg i.m., i.v. stat
Ethosuximide	500 mg daily o initially	Under 6 yr: 250 mg D o
Fenbufen	600 mg D o	Not in children
Fenoprofen	200 mg q.d.s. o	Not in children
Flavoxate	200 mg t.d.s. o	Not in children
Flecainide	100–200 mg b.d. o **a** 2 mg/kg 20 min I up to 150 mg **b** 1.5 mg/kg I 1 h **c** 250 µg/kg/h	
Fludrocortisone	Replacement: 0.1–0.3 mg/day o Hyperplasia: 1–2 mg/day o	Dose adjusted to weight, age and clinical condition
Flumazenil	200 µg i.v. Repeat 15 s up to 500 µg initially Max. 2 mg Infusion: 100–400 µg/h	
Flunitrazepam	0.5–1 mg *nocte* o	Not in children
Fluphenazine	6.25–12.5 mg i.m. initially	Not in children
Flurazepam	15–30 mg *nocte* o	
Folic acid	10–20 mg daily o 5 mg D i.v.	5–15 mg D o
Folinate calcium	15 mg D o 3 mg D i.v. Increase dose with methotrexate, see manufacturer's data sheet	0.25 mg/kg/day o
Frusemide	20–80 mg o, i.m., i.v. High dose (250–500 mg) See manufacturer's data sheet	1–3 mg/kg o 0.5–1.5 mg/kg i.m., i.v.
Furosemide	See Frusemide	
Glibenclamide	5 mg daily o initially Max. 15 mg	
Gliclazide	40–80 mg D o initially	
Glipizide	2.5–5 mg D o initially	
Gliquidone	15 mg D o initially	
Glymidine	1–1.5 mg D o initially	
Glucagon	0.5–1 u s.c., i.m., i.v.	As adult

Drug	Adult dose	Paediatric dose
Glyceryl trinitrate (Also see Section 6.5)	GTN-1 tab subling. p.r.n. Sustac: 2.5 mg t.d.s. initially Nitrolingual: metered spray o Percutol: 1–2 in percut. 4 h 10–200 µg/min I i.v.	
Glycopyrrolate	0.2–0.4 mg i.m., i.v. 1–4 mg b.d. oral.	0.004–0.008 mg/kg i.m., i.v. Max. 0.2 mg
Guanethidine	20 mg D o 2–10 mg i.m.	
Haloperidol	0.5–5 mg b.d. o 10–20 mg i.m.	0.05 mg/kg/day o Not parenteral
Heparin	Load: 5000 units i.v. 10 000 units 6 h by infusion or i.v. injection. Thrombosis prophylaxis: 5000 units s.c. 12 h	
Hyaluronidase	1500 units s.c., i.m.	
Hydralazine	25 mg b.d., t.d.s. o	
Hydrochlorothiazide	20–40 mg i.v. slowly	
Hydrocortisone	20–30 mg D o 100 mg 6 h i.m. for post- operative sterioid cover 100–500 mg 6 h i.v.	Up to 1 yr: 25 mg 1–5 yr: 50 mg 6–12 yr: 100 mg or 5–50 mg/kg/day
Hydroxyzine	25–100 mg t.d.s. o	Up to 6 yr: 30–50 mg/day DD o
Hyoscine	0.3–0.6 mg s.c. o 0.4 mg i.m.	0.008 mg/kg i.m. 3–5 yr: 0.075–0.1 mg o 6–12 yr: 0.1–0.3 mg o
Imipramine	25 mg b.d. o initially	Enuresis only
Indoramin	25 mg b.d. o initially	
Inositol	1 g t.d.s. o	
Insulin	See section on diabetes p. 149	
Ipratroprium	Metered inhaler Ventilator nebulizer: 0.1–0.5 mg q.d.s.	Ventilator nebulizer: Over 3 yr: 0.1–0.5 mg t.d.s.
Iproniazid	100–150 mg D o, then reduce to 25–50 mg/day	Not in children
Isocarboxazid	10–30 mg D o	Not in children
Isoprenaline (Also see Section 6.5)	Sustained release tab: 30 mg 8 h o initially Infusion i.v. 1 mg in 100 ml or higher conc. Stat i.v. dose: 10–20 µg	

11

Drug	Adult dose	Paediatric dose
Isosorbide	5–10 mg subling. 10–30 mg q.d.s. o Infusion: 2–10 mg h i.v.	Not in children
Labetalol	100–200 mg b.d. o 10–20 mg i.v. Repeat depending on effect. Infusion: 1 mg/ml. Rate depends on effect.	
Lactulose	Hepatic encephalopathy: 30–50 ml syrup t.d.s.	
Lanatoside C	Load dose: 0.8–1.6 mg i.m., i.v., over 24 h. 0.25–1.5 mg/day o	0.02–0.04 mg/kg i.v. then 0.01–0.03 mg/kg/day 3DD o
Levorphanol	1.5–4.5 mg b.d. o 2–4 mg s.c., i.m. 1–2 mg i.v.	Not in children
Lignocaine	100 mg i.v. stat Infusion: 1–2 mg/min i.v. See also anaesthetic section, p. 26	
Loperamide	2 tabs initially. Then 1 tab after loose stool Max. 8 tab/day	Syrup: 1 mg/5 ml 4–8 yr: 5 ml q.d.s. o 9–12 yr: 10 ml q.d.s. o
Lorazepam	1–4 mg o 0.025–0.05 mg/kg i.m., i.v.	Not in children
Lormetazepam	0.5–1 mg *nocte* o	Not in children
Medazepam	5 mg b.d., t.d.s. o 10–15 mg o *nocte*	1–1.5 mg/kg/day o
Medigoxin	Load: 0.2 mg b.d. o, i.v. –3 days Maintain: 0.1 mg b.d. D	0.01 mg/kg 6 h 2–4 doses 0.01 mg/kg/day
Mefanamic acid	500 mg t.d.s. o	Suspension: 50 mg/5 ml Over 6 months: 25 mg/kg/day DD
Menadiol	10 mg D o 10 mg i.m.	5 mg D o
Meprobamate	400 mg t.d.s. o	
Meptazinol	75–100 mg 2–4 h i.m. 50–100 mg 2–4 h i.v.	Not in children
Mepyramine	100 mg t.d.s. o initially	Up to 3 yr: 12.5–25 mg t.d.s. o 3–7 yr: 25–50 mg t.d.s. 7–14 yr: 25–75 mg t.d.s.
Metaraminol	5 mg i.m., 1 mg i.v.	
Metformin	500 mg 8 h o	

Drug	Adult dose	Paediatric dose
Methadone	5–10 mg o, s.c., i.m., i.v.	Not in children
Methoxamine	5 mg i.m., i.v.	
Methyldopa	250 mg b.d. t.d.s. o initially 250–500 mg 6 h i.v.	10 mg/kg/day 2–4DD o 20–40 mg/kg/day 4DD i.v.
Methylene blue	75–100 mg i.v. (1% soln.)	
Methylphenidate	10–15 mg b.d. o 10–20 mg s.c., i.m. i.v.	Over 6 yr: 5–10 mg t.d.s. o Not parenteral
Methylprednisolone	Oral dose variable 16–40 mg/day, see manufacturer's data sheet High dose i.v.: 30 mg/kg 6 h	
Metoclopramide	5–10 mg o, i.m., i.v.	Liquid prep: 1 mg/ml Up to 1 yr: 1 mg b.d. o, i.m. 3–5 yr: 2 mg b.d. o, i.m. 6–14 yr: 2.5–5 mg t.d.s. o, i.m. Max. dose: 0.5 mg/kg/day
Metroprolol	50 mg b.d. o initially 5 mg i.v. slowly. Repeat up to 15 mg	
Mexilitene	Load: 400 mg, then 200 mg t.d.s. or q.d.s. o 100–250 mg i.v. slowly. Infusion: 250 mg in 500 ml 0.5 mg (1 ml)/min	
Midazolam	0.07 mg/kg i.v., i.m.	
Minoxidil	5 mg D o initially	0.2 mg/kg/day o Max. 1 mg/kg/day
Mithramycin	See Plicamycin	
Morphine	10–15 mg 4–6 h o, s.c., i.m. 5 mg i.v. Extradural and intrathecal: 2–4 mg *Preservative free* morphine *CAUTION: RESPIRATORY* *DEPRESSION*	0.2 mg/kg i.m. 0.1 mg/kg i.v.
Nadolol	Angina: 40 mg/day o initially Hyperten: 80 mg/day o	
Naloxone	0.1–0.4 mg s.c., i.m., i.v.	0.01 mg/kg i.m., i.v.
Nandrolone	25–50 mg/week i.m.	Max. 1 mg/kg/month i.m.
Nefopam	30–60 mg t.d.s. o 20 mg 6 h i.m.	Not in children

11

Drug	Adult dose	Paediatric dose
Neostigmine	75–300 mg daily DD o 1–2.5 mg/day DD s.c., i.m. i.v.	*Oral:* Neonate: 1–5 mg 4 h o Child: 15–60 mg/day DD o *Parenteral:* Neonate: 50–250 µg 4 h Child: 200–500 µg/day DD
	See also anaesthetic section, p. 14	
Nicardipine	30 mg t.d.s. o initially	
Nicotinyl alcohol	25–50 mg q.d.s. o	Not in children
Nicoumalone	1st day 8–12 mg o 2nd day 4–8 mg o Then as per prothrombin ratio	
Nifedipine	10–20 mg t.d.s. o	
Nikethamide	0.5–1 g i.v.	
Nitrazepam	5–10 mg *nocte* o	2.5–5 mg o
Nitroprusside (Also see Section 6.5)	50 mg in 500 ml 5% Dextrose Infusion to control hyper- tension. Use drip counter and burette *Monitor carefully* Higher concentrations used in ITU (50 mg/100 ml)	
Nizatidine	300 mg *nocte* o	
Noradrenaline (Also see Section 6.5)	1 mg in 100 ml 5% Dextrose: rate depends on response	
Nortriptyline	10 mg q.d.s. o	Enuresis only
Orciprenaline	1. 20 mg q.d.s. o 2. Metered aerosol 3. 0.2 ml, 5% soln. in 2 ml by nebulizer 4. 0.5 mg i.m.	See manufacturer's data sheet
Orphenadrine	50 mg t.d.s. o initially 20–40 mg i.m.	
Oxprenolol	Angina: 40–160 mg t.d.s. o Hyperten: 80 mg b.d. o 2 mg i.m., i.v. slowly Increments up to 16 mg	
Oxytocin	By infusion: 1 unit/l $1\frac{1}{2}$–3 mu/min	
Papaveretum	10–20 mg 4 h i.m. 2.5 mg i.v.	0.4 mg/kg i.m.

Drug	Adult dose	Paediatric dose
Paracetamol	1 g q.d.s. o	Elixir: 120 mg/5 ml 6 months–1 yr: 2.5–5 ml 1–6 yr: 5–10 ml 6–12 yr: 10–20 ml Max. 4 doses in 24 h
Paraldehyde	5–10 ml. i.m.	Intramuscular doses: Up to 6 months: 0.5 ml 6–12 months: 1 ml 1–2 yr: 1.5 ml 3–5 yr: 3 ml 6–12 yr: 5 ml
Penicillamine	Adult and paediatric dosage complex: see manufacturer's data sheet	
Pentaerythritol	30–60 mg t.d.s. o	
Pentazocine	30–60 mg 4–6 h s.c., i.m., i.v. 50–100 mg 4 h o 50 mg rect. suppository q.d.s.	6–12 yr: 25 mg 4 h o Max. 1 mg/kg i.m. 0.5 mg/kg i.v.
Pentolinium	Up to 10 mg i.v. in 0.5 mg increments	
Perphenazine	4 mg t.d.s. o 5 mg 6 h i.m.	Not in children
Pethidine	50–100 mg 4 h i.m. 10–20 mg i.v. or by infusion 50–150 mg 4 h o	1 mg/kg o 0.5–2 mg/kg o
Phenazocine	5 mg 4–6 h o Max. single dose 20 mg	Not in children
Phenindione	1st day: 200 mg o 2nd day: 100 mg o Then adjust to prothrombin ratio	
Phenobarbitone	30–60 mg t.d.s. o, i.m. 100–200 mg as hypnotic	Up to 1 year: 15–30 mg/day 1–2 years: 30–60 mg/day
Phenoperidine	1–2 mg i.v. This drug is usually administered during assisted ventilation	0.1–0.15 mg/kg i.v.
Phenoxybenzamine	10 mg b.d. o initially 1 mg/kg i.v. very slowly	1–2 mg/kg/day o 1 mg/kg i.v.
Phentolamine	Up to 10 mg i.v. in 1 mg increments Infusion: 10 mg in 100 ml, adjust rate for effect	

11

Drug	Adult dose	Paediatric dose
Phenylbutazone	200 mg t.d.s. o, initially Then 100 mg t.d.s. o 250 mg *nocte* rect. supp.	5–10 mg/kg/day DD o
Phenylephrine	1.Topical nasal spray 2.100 μg i.v. 3.Infusion: 10 mg in 100 ml Adjust rate for effect	
Phenytoin	Epilepsy: 100 mg b.d.– q.d.s. o 150–200 mg i.v. slowly or i.m. Arrhythmias: 3.5–5 mg/kg i.v.	See manufacturer's data sheet
Physostigmine	0.2–2 mg i.m., i.v.	Up to 0.03 mg/kg
Pindolol	2.5–5 mg t.d.s. o	
Piroxicam	20 mg D o	Not in children
Plicamycin	25 μg/kg/day i.v. Infusion: over 6 h in 1000 ml 5% dextrose See manufacturer's data sheet	
Poldine	2 mg q.d.s. o	
Prazosin	0.5 mg b.d. or t.d.s. o initially	
Prednisolone	Dosage very variable see manufacturer's data sheet	
Prenalterol	2.5 mg i.v. slowly. Infusion: 0.5 mg/min	
Primidone	125 mg D o initially	See manufacturer's data sheet
Probenicid	250 b.d. o initially	Over 2 yr: 25 mg/kg 4 DD o initially
Procainamide	250 mg 6 h o 25 mg/min i.v. Max. 1 g	
Prochlorperazine	5 mg t.d.s. o 12.5 mg i.m.	Syrup: 5 mg in 5 ml 1–5 yr: 2.5 ml b.d. o 6–12 yr: 5 ml b.d. or t.d.s. o
Procyclidine	2.5 mg t.d.s. o 5–10 mg i.v.	
Promazine	25–100 mg t.d.s. o 50 mg 6 h i.m., i.v.	25 mg i.m. or proportional to adult dose
Promethazine	25–50 mg o, i.m.	Elixir: 5 mg in 5 ml As sedative 6 months–1 yr: 10 mg 1–5 yr: 15–20 mg 5–10 yr: 20–25 mg i.m.: 5–10 yr 6.25–12.5 mg

Drug	Adult dose	Paediatric dose
Propanolol	10–40 mg t.d.s. o 1–2 mg i.v.	0.25–1 mg/kg t.d.s. o 0.025–0.1 mg/kg i.v.
Propantheline	15–30 mg 8 h o, i.v.	2 mg/kg/day DD max.
Protamine	1 mg neutralizes 1 mg (100 units) of heparin Usual dose about 3 mg/kg	As adult
Protryptiline	10 mg t.d.s. o initially	
Pseudoephrine	60 mg t.d.s. o	Elixir: 30 mg in 5 ml 3–12 months: 2.5 ml t.d.s. o 1–6 yr: 5 ml t.d.s. o 6–12 yr: 7.5 ml t.d.s. o
Pyridostigmine	300 mg–1.2 g daily DD o	Neonate: 5–10 mg 4 h o Child: 10 mg o initially Parenteral: Neonate: 0.2–0.4 mg 4 h i.m. Child: 0.25–1 mg i.m. initially
Quinalbarbitone	50–100 mg *nocte* o 200–300 mg o for premed.	Sedation: 50–100 mg o
Quinidine	200–400 mg b.d. o	
Ranitidine	150 mg b.d. o 50 mg 6–8 h i.v.	
Salbutamol	1. 4 mg q.d.s. o 2. 0.5 mg 4 h s.c., i.m. 3. 0.25 mg i.v. slowly 4. 3–20 µg/min i.v. infusion 5. 5–10 mg of nebulized respirator soln. 6. Metered aerosol	1. Oral syrup 2 mg in 5 ml 2–6 yr: 2–5–5 ml t.d.s. 6–12 yr: 5 ml t.d.s. 2. 2.5 mg nebulized 3. Metered aerosol 4. Not parenteral
Sotalol	80 mg b.d. o, initially 10–20 mg i.v. slowly	
Spironolactone	100–200 mg D o	3 mg/kg/day DD o
Stanozolol	5 mg D o 50 mg i.m. 2–3 weekly	Under 6 yr: 2.5 mg D o 6–10 yr: 2.5–5 mg D o
Streptokinase	600 000 i.u. over 30 min i.v. 100 000 i.u. i.v. h for 3 days	See manufacturer's data sheet
Sulindac	200 mg b.d. o	Not in children
Sulphasalazine	500 mg b.d.–q.d.s. o	Reduce dose per body weight
Temazepam	10–30 mg o	
Terbutaline	5 mg b.d. o 0.25–0.5 mg q.d.s. s.c., i.m., i.v. slowly. Metered aerosol Ventilator nebulizer: 2–5 mg	Syrup: 0.3 mg/ml 3–7 yr: 2.5–5 ml 8 h o 7–15 yr: 5–10 ml 8 h o Parenteral: 0.01 mg/kg s.c., i.m., i.v. Max. 0.3 mg

11

Drug	Adult dose	Paediatric dose
Theophylline	Several preparations with variable dosage See manufacturer's data sheet	
Thiethylperazine	10 mg t.d.s. o 6.5 mg i.m. 6.5 mg rect.	Not under 15 yr
Thymoxamine	40 mg q.d.s. o 0.1 mg/kg q.d.s. i.v.	Not in children
Thyroxine	50–100 μg D o	Infant: 25 μg/day then reduce Child: 2.5–5 μg/kg/day o
Timolol	10 mg daily o	
Tocainide	400 mg t.d.s. o 500–750 mg i.v. slowly or infusion	
Tolazamide	100–250 mg D o initially	
Tolbutamide	1st day–3 g o 2nd day–2 g o Maintain 1–1.5 g D o	Not in children
Tranexamic acid	1.5 g t.d.s. o 500 mg–1 g i.v.	25 mg/kg/dose o 10 mg/kg/dose i.v.
Triamcinolone	Up to 24 mg/day DD o	
Triamterene	150–250 mg/day o	Not in children
Triazolam	0.25 mg *nocte* o	
Triclofos	1–2 g *nocte* o	Up to 1 yr: 100–250 mg o 1–5 yr: 250–500 mg o 6–12 yr: 500 mg–1 g o
Trifluoperazine	2–10 mg/day DD o 1 mg i.m.	Syrup: 1 mg in 5 ml 3–5 yr: 1 mg/day DD o 6–12 yr: 4 mg/day DD o
Trimeprazine	10 mg t.d.s. o	2.5–5 mg t.d.s. o Premed: 2–4 mg/kg o
Trimetaphan	250 mg in 500 ml 5% dextrose Infusion as required	
Trimipramine	50–75 mg *nocte* o	Not in children
Triprolidine	2.5–5 mg t.d.s. o	Elixir: 2 mg in 5 ml Up to 1 yr: 2.5 ml t.d.s. o 1–6 yr: 5 ml t.d.s. o 6–12 yr: 7.5 ml t.d.s. o
Urokinase	Load: 4400 i.u./kg in 10 min Then 4400 i.u./kg/h, infusion for 12 h	
Valproate sodium	600 mg/day o, initially Up to 10 mg/kg i.v. Infusion: up to 2.5 g/day	Over 20 kg: 400 mg/day o Under 20 kg: 20 mg/kg/day o 20–30 mg/kg/day i.v.

Drug	Adult dose	Paediatric dose
Vasopressin	5–20 units b.d. s.c., i.m.	
Verapamil	40–120 mg t.d.s. o 10 mg i.v. slowly and repeat 5 mg. Infusion: 5–10 mg/h Max. 100 mg/24 h	10 mg/kg/day DD o *Intravenous:* Infant: 0.75–2 mg 1–5 yr: 2–3 mg 6–15 yr: 2.5–5 mg
Vitamin K	10 mg i.v.	1 mg i.m., i.v.
Warfarin	10 mg, 5 mg, 5 mg, on days 1, 2 and 3, then maintain on PTI Reduce dose according to weight, age and liver function	

11.2 Antibiotics

11.2.1 Introduction

This section on antibiotics is not a comprehensive guide to all aspects of antibacterial therapy. It covers only those antibiotics used for intensive therapy and other emergency situations in hospital. Oral and parenteral doses are included in separate tables. The information is basic and sufficient to initiate therapy safely. It is not intended to replace the more detailed information available from the manufacturer's data sheet.

11.2.2 Antibiotic dose tables

The following tables show the adult and paediatric doses of the antibiotics in common use in hospital. These doses are the normal range and unless the infection is severe the lower end of the range should be used initially. The tables are intended for reference and initiation of therapy in the absence of the manufacturer's data sheet. In severe infections much higher doses can often be used, but in these circumstances it is wise to consult a microbiologist for advice.

11

Paediatric doses

These are usually given as mg/kg/day when the total 24 h dose must be divided up as indicated. In some instances, the dose given

is that actually administered at the intervals indicated.
All paediatric doses must be carefully checked before prescribing.

Renal function
Most antibiotics must be given in reduced dose in the presence of any degree of renal failure, if possible, blood levels should be monitored frequently.

A detailed guide to drug therapy in renal failure can be found in the manufacturers' data sheets and in the *British National Formulary.*

Infusions
Detailed information about dilution and infusion of antibiotics can be found in the manufacturers' data sheets or in the *British National Formulary.*

11.2.3 Oral doses of antibiotics

Antibiotic	Adult oral dose	Paediatric oral dose
Acyclovir	200 mg 5 times D (immunocompromized 400 mg)	<2 yr $\frac{1}{2}$ adult dose >2 yr adult dose
Amoxycillin	250–500 mg 8 h	125 mg 8 h
Amphotericin	100–200 mg 6 h (tab) 10 mg q.d.s. (lozenges)	1 ml (100 mg) q.d.s. (suspension)
Ampicillin	250 mg–1 g 6 h	125 mg 6 h
Carfecillin	0.5–1 g t.d.s. o	
Cefaclor	250 mg 8 h	20 mg/kg/day DD, 8 h
Cephalexin	250–500 mg 6 h	25–50 mg/kg/day DD, 6 h
Cephradine	250–500 mg 6 h	25–50 mg/kg/day DD, 6 h
Chloramphenicol	500 mg 6 h	
Ciprofloxacin	250–750 mg b.d. o	See manufacturer's data sheet
Cloxacillin	500 mg 6 h	$\frac{1}{4}$–$\frac{1}{2}$ adult dose
Colistin	1.5–3 million units 8 h	Up to 15 kg: 250 000–500 000 units 8 h 15–30 kg: 750 000–1 500 000 units 8 h
Co-trimoxazole	960 mg (2 tab) 12 h	Paediatric suspension: 240 mg in 5 ml 6 weeks–6 months: 2.5 ml b.d. 6 months–6 years: 5 ml b.d. 6–12 yr: 10 ml b.d.
Doxycycline	200 mg 1st day 100 mg D	

Antibiotic	Adult oral dose	Paediatric oral dose
Erythromycin	250–500 mg 6 h	125–250 mg 6 h
Ethambutol	15 mg/kg/day	25 mg/kg/day (reduce to 15 mg after 60 days) (see manufacturer's data sheet)
Flucloxacillin	250 mg 6 h	Under 2 yr: $\frac{1}{4}$ adult dose 2–10 yr: $\frac{1}{2}$ adult dose
Flucytosine	150–200 mg/kg/day 4DD	As adult
Isoniazid	3 mg/kg/day (max. 300 mg)	6 mg/kg/day
Kanamycin	250–500 mg 6 h	Reduce dose according to age and weight
Ketoconazole	200 mg D	3 mg/kg/day
Metronidazole	Oral: 400 mg 8 h Rectal: 1 g 8 h	7.5 mg/kg 8 h
Miconazole	250 mg 6 h	
Nalidixic acid	1 g 6 h	Over 3 months: 50 mg/kg/day DD
Neomycin	1 g 4 h	
Nitrofurantoin	100 mg 6 h	Suspension: 25 mg/5 ml 3–30 months: 2.5 ml q.d.s. $2\frac{1}{2}$–6 yr: 5 ml q.d.s. 6–11 yr: 10 ml q.d.s. 11–14 yr: 15 ml q.d.s.
Nystatin	500 000 units 6 h (tab) 100 000 units 6 h (oral susp.)	Oral susp: 100 000 units 1 ml) 6 h
Phenoxymethyl- penicillin	250–500 mg 6 h	$\frac{1}{4}$–$\frac{1}{2}$ adult dose
Pyrazinamide	20–35 mg/kg/day 3DD	Not in children
Rifampicin	600 mg D (10 mg/kg/day)	Up to 20 mg/kg/day (max. 600 mg/day)
Sodium fusidate	500 mg 8 h	Suspension: 175 mg/5 ml 0–1 yr: 1 ml/kg/day 3DD 1–5 yr: 5 ml t.d.s. 5–12 yr: 10 ml t.d.s.
Sulphamethizole	200 mg 5 times per day	0–5 yr: 50 mg × 5 D 6–12 yr: 100 mg × 5 D
Tetracycline	250–500 mg 6 h	Not in children
Tinidazole	2 g 1st day 1 g D thereafter	Not in children under 12 yr
Trimethoprim	200 mg 12 h	2–5 months: 25 mg b.d. 6 months–5 yr: 50 mg b.d. 6–12 yr: 100 mg b.d.
Vancomycin	500 mg 6 h	44 mg/kg/day DD

11

11.2.4 Parenteral doses of antibiotics

Antibiotic	Adult parenteral dose	Paediatric parenteral dose
Acyclovir	5 mg/kg 8 h i.v. over 1 h	As adult
Amikacin	15 mg/kg/day 2DD i.m., i.v. B, I	As adult
Amoxycillin	500 mg 8 h i.m. 1 g 6 h i.v. B, I	50–100 mg/kg/day DD i.m., i.v.
Amphotericin	0.25 mg/kg/day DD i.v. I initially	As adult
Ampicillin	500 mg 6 h i.m., i.v. B, I	$\frac{1}{2}$ adult dose
Azlocillin	Bolus i.v.: 2 g 8 h Infusion: 5 g 8 h	See manufacturer's data sheet
Aztreonam	1 g i.m., i.v. B, I	
Benethamine penicillin	1 ampoule every 3 days i.m.	0–6 yr: $\frac{1}{4}$ ampoule i.m. 7–12 yr: $\frac{1}{2}$ ampoule i.m.
Benzylpenicillin	600 mg 6 h i.m. Up to 24 g D by infusion See manufacturer's data sheet	Neonate: 30 mg/kg/day DD, i.m. Up to 12 yr: 20 mg/kg/day DD i.m.
Carbenicillin	2 g 6 h i.m. 5 g 6 h i.v. B, I	50–100 mg/kg/day 4DD i.m. 250–400 mg/kg/day 4DD i.v. B, I
Cefotaxime	1 g 12 h i.m., i.v. B,I	100–150 mg/kg/day 4DD, i.m., i.v.
Cefoxitin	1–2 g 8 h i.m., i.v. B,I. See manufacturer's data sheet	Over 3 months: 80–160 mg/kg/day 4DD i.m., i.v.
Cefsulodin	1–4 g/day 4DD i.m., i.v. B, I	20–40 mg/kg/day DD
Ceftazidime	1–6 g/day DD i.v., i.m.	
Ceftizoxime	1–2 g 8–12 h, i.v., i.m.	Over 3 months 30–60 mg/kg/day 2–4 DD i.v., i.m.
Cefuroxime	750 mg 8 h i.m., i.v. B.	30–100 mg/kg/day 3 DD
Cephamandole	500 mg–2 g 4–8 h i.m., i.v. B,I.	50–100 mg/kg/day 4 DD
Cephazolin	500 mg–1 g 6–12 h i.m., i.v. B,I.	25–50 mg/kg/day 4 DD
Cephradine	500 mg–1 g 6 h i.m., i.v. B,I	50–100 mg/kg/day 4 DD
Chloramphenicol	i.m. possible but not recommended 1 g 6–8 h i.v. B,I	Infant: 25 mg/kg/day 4 DD Child: 50 mg/kg/day 4DD
Ciprofloxacin	200 mg 12 h i.v., I	

Antibiotic	Adult parenteral dose	Paediatric parenteral dose
Cloxacillin	250 mg 6 h i.m. 500 mg 5 h i.v. B,I.	$\frac{1}{4}-\frac{1}{2}$ adult dose
Colistin	2 million units 8 h i.m., i.v. B,I.	50 000 u/kg/day 3 DD
Co-trimoxazole	960 mg (1 ampoule) 12 h i.m. 960 mg (2 ampoules) 12 h i.v. infusion *Caution: special preparations for i.m. and i.v. use should not be confused*	
Erythromycin	Not i.m. 500 mg 8 h i.v. B,I	30–50 mg/kg/day 4 DD i.v. B,I
Flucloxacillin	250 mg 6 h i.m. 250–500 mg i.v. B,I	$\frac{1}{4}-\frac{1}{2}$ adult dose
Flucytosine	150–200 mg/kg/day 4DD i.v. I	As adult
Gentamicin	80 mg 8 h i.m., i.v. B,I, or 2–5 mg/kg daily DD 8 h i.v., i.m.	Infant: 3 mg/kg 12 h i.m., i.v. Child: 2 mg/kg 8 h i.m., i.v.
Imipenem	1–2 g daily 3–4 DD i.v., I Max. 50 mg/kg/day or 4 g	See manufacturer's data sheet
Isoniazid	3 mg/kg/day i.m. (max. 300 mg) (TB meningitis: 10 mg/kg/day)	6 mg/kg/day i.m.
Kanamycin	250 mg 6 h i.m. 15–30 mg/kg/day 2 DD i.v. I	15 mg/kg/day 2–4 DD i.m. 15–30 mg/kg/day 2–3 DD i.v. I
Latamoxef	250 mg–3 g 12 h i.m., i.v. B,I	Infant: 25 mg/kg 12 h Child: 50 mg/kg 12 h i.m., i.v.
Mecillinam	5–15 mg/kg 6–8 h i.m., i.v., B,I	
Methicillin	1 g 4–6 h i.m., i.v. B,I	Under 2 yr: $\frac{1}{4}$ adult dose 2–10 yr: $\frac{1}{2}$ adult dose
Metronidazole	500 mg 8 h i.v. I. Rectal: 1 g 8 h	7.5 mg/kg/ 8 h rect., i.v.
Mezlocillin	500 mg–2 g 6–8 h i.m. (i.v. if poss.) Bolus: 2 g 6–8 h i.v. Infusion: 5 g 6–8 h i.v.	See manufacturer's data sheet
Miconazole	600 mg 8 h i.v. I	40 mg/kg/day DD

Netilmicin	4–6 mg/kg/day DD 12 h i.m.,
	  i.v. B,I
		Neonate: 6 mg/kg/day DD
		  12 h
		Infant: 7.5–9 mg/kg/day DD
		  12 h
		Child: 6–7.5 mg/kg/day DD
		  12 h

11

Antibiotic	Adult parenteral dose	Paediatric parenteral dose
Piperacillin	100–150 mg/kg/day 4DD i.m., i.v. B,I	Infant: 100–300 mg/kg/day 2DD Child: 100–300 mg/kg/day 3DD
Procaine penicillin	300 mg 12 h i.m.	Reduce dose proportionally under 25 kg
Rifampicin	In severe infections an intravenous preparation is available at special request	
Sodium fusidate	500 mg infusion over 6 h at 8 h intervals	Under 50 kg: 6–7 mg/kg 8 h by infusion i.v. over 6 h
Streptomycin	1 g D i.m. (750 mg over 40 yr)	30 mg/kg D i.m. (max. 1 g)
Tetracycline	100 mg 8 h i.m. 500 mg 12 h i.v. I	Not in children
Ticarcillin	15–20 g/day 4DD i.m., i.v. B,I	200–300 mg/kg/day 4DD
Tinidazole	800 mg D i.v. I	Not in children
Tobramycin	3–5 mg/kg/day DD 8 h i.m., i.v. B,I	Infant: 4 mg/kg/day DD 12 h Child: 6 mg/kg/day DD 6 h
Trimethoprim	150–250 mg 12 h i.v. B,I	Under 12 yr: 8 mg/kg/day 3DD i.v.
Vancomycin	500 mg 6 h i.v. I	44 mg/kg/day 4 DD i.v. I

11.2.5 Therapeutic levels of some antibiotics

Drug	Trough level	Peak level
Amikacin	< 5 mg/l	15–30 mg/l
Chloramphenicol	< 8–10 mg/l	Up to 25 mg/l
Flucytosine	40–70 µg/l	> 120 µg/l (toxic)
Gentamicin	< 2 mg/l	5–10 mg/l
Kanamycin	< 5 mg/l	15–25 mg/l
Tobramycin	< 2 mg/l	5–10 mg/l
Vancomycin	< 5–10 mg/l	20–30mg/l

11.3 Brand names and pharmacopoeal names conversion table with main use indicator (see key on pp. 211–212)

Brand name	Pharmacopoeal name	Main use	Brand name	Pharmacopoeal name	Main use
Acepril	Captopril	Hypot.	Alloferin	Alcuronium	Anaes.
Actal	Alexitol	Gastr.	Aloral	Allopurinol	Gout
Acthar	ACTH	Hormo.	Alunex	Chlorpheniramine	Aller.
Actidil	Triprolidine	Aller.	Alupent	Metaproterenol	Asthm.
Actifed	Trypolikine	Aller.	Alupent	Orciprenaline	Asthm.
Acupan	Nefopam	Analg.	Aluzine	Frusemide	Diure.
Adalat	Nifedipine	Arrhy.	Amicar	Aminocaproic acid	Haema.
Adapin	Doxepin	Psych.	Amilco	Amiloride/thiazide	Diure.
Adriamycin	Doxorubicin	Neopl.	Amiline	Amitriptyline	Psych.
Aerolate	Theophylline	Asthm.	Amisec	Aminophylline	Asthm.
Afrinol	Pseudoephedrine	Aller.	Amitid	Amitriptyline	Psych.
Akineton	Biperiden	Parki.	Amsidine	Amsacrine	Neopl.
Alcobon	Flucytosine	Neopl.	Amytal	Amylobarbitone	Hypno.
Alcopar	Bephenium	Micro.	Anafranil	Clomipramine	Psych.
Aldactide	Spironolactone/thiazide	Diure.	Anapolon	Oxymetholone	Haema.
Aldactone	Spironolactone	Diure.	Ancoloxin	Meclozine	N/V
Aldomet	Methyl DOPA	Hypot.	Anectine	Suxamethonium	Anaes
Alevaire	Tyloxapol	Respi.	Angilol	Propanolol	Betab.
Algodex	Propoxyphene	Analg.	Anquil	Benperidol	Anxio.
Alkeran	Melphalan	Neopl.	Ansolysen	Pentolinium	Hypot.
Allegron	Nortryptiline	Psych.	Antabuse	Disulphiram	Alcoh.

11

Brand name	Pharmacopoeal name	Main use
Anthisan	Mepyramine	Hista.
Antilirium	Physostigmine	Anaes.
Antipress	Imipramine	Psych.
Anturan	Sulphinpyrazone	Gout
Apisate	Diethylproprion	Metab.
Apresoline	Hydrallazine	Hypot.
Aprinox	Bendrofluazide	Diure.
Apsifen	Ibuprofen	NSAID
Apsolol	Propanolol	Betab.
Apsolox	Oxprenolol	Betab.
Aquastat	Benzthiazide	Diure.
Aralen	Chloroquine	Micro.
Aramine	Metaraminol	Hypot.
Arfonad	Trimetaphan	Hypot.
Aristogel	Triamcinolone	Stero.
Arpicolin	Procyclidine	Parki.
Artane	Benzhexol	Parki
Artracin	Indomethacin	NSAID
Arvin	Ancrod	Haema.
Asendin	Amoxapine	Psych.
Asmaven	Salbutamol	Asthm.
Aspav	Aspirin/papaveretum	Analg.
Atarax	Hydroxyzine	Anxio.
Ativan	Lorazepam	Anxio.

Brand name	Pharmacopoeal name	Main use
Atromid-S	Clofibrate	Metab.
Atrovent	Ipratropium	Asthm.
Aventyl	Nortryptyline	Psych.
Avloclor	Chloroquine	Micro.
Avomine	Promethazine	Anxio.
Azamune	Azathioprine	Neopl.
Azolid	Phenylbutazone	NSAID
Banlin	Propantheline	Gut
Baratol	Indoramin	Betab.
Beconase	Beclomethasone	Stero.
Becotide	Beclomethasone	Stero.
Benadryl	Diphenhydramine	Hista.
Bendogen	Bethanidine	Hypot.
Bendylate	Diphenhydramine	Hista.
Benemid	Probenecid	Gout
Benoral	Benorylate	Arthr.
Bentex	Benzhexol	Parki.
Bentyl	Dicyclomine	Muscu.
Benztrone	Oestradiol	Hormo.
Berkaprine	Azathioprine	Neopl.
Berkatens	Verapamil	Arrhy.
Berkdopa	Levodopa	Parki.
Berkfurin	Nitrofurantoin	Antib.
Berkolol	Propanolol	Betab.

Brand name	Pharmacopoeal name	Main use	Brand name	Pharmacopoeal name	Main use
Berkozide	Bendrofluazide	Diure.	Buscopan	Hyoscine	N/V
Berotec	Fenoterol	Asthm.	Butacote	Phenylbutazone	NSAID
Beta-Cardone	Sotalol	Betab.	Butazolidine	Phenylbutazone	NSAID
Betaloc	Metoprolol	Betab.	Cafergot	Ergotamine + caffeine	Migra.
Betim	Timolol	Eyes	Calan	Verapamil	Arrhy.
Betnesol	Betamethasone	Stero.	Calciparine	Heparin	Haema.
Betoptic	Betaxolol	Betab.	Calcitare	Calcitonin	Paget.
Bextasol	Betamethasone	Stero.	Calpol	Paracetamol	Analg.
Bezalip	Bezafibrate	Metab.	Camolit	Lithium	Psych.
Biogastrone	Carbenoxalone	Gastr.	Caplenal	Allopurinol	Gout
Biophylline	Theophylline	Asthm.	Capoten	Captopril	Hypot.
Bisolvon	Bromhexine	Resp.	Caprin	Aspirin	Analg.
Blocadren	Timolol	Glauc.	Carbacel	Carbachol	Choli.
Bolvidon	Mianserin	Psych.	Cardene	Nicardipine	Arrhy.
Bradilan	Nicofuranose	Vascu.	Cardiacap	Pentaerythritol	Arrhy.
Bretylate	Bretylium tosilate	Arrhy.	Cardilate	Erythrityl tetranitrate	Arrhy.
Brevidil-M	Suxamethonium	Anaes.	Cardioquin	Quinidine	Arrhy.
Bricanyl	Terbutaline	Respi.	Catapres	Clonidine	Hypot.
Brietal	Methohexitone	Anaes.	Cedinalid	Lanatoside-C	Arrhy.
Brocadopa	Levodopa	Parki.	Cedocard	Isosorbide	Arrhy.
Broflex	Benzhexol	Parki.	Celestone	Betamethasone	Stero.
Bronchodil	Reproterol	Asthm.	Centyl	Bendrofluazide	Diure.
Brufen	Ibuprofen	NSAID	Cerebid	Papaverine	Vascu.
Burinex	Bumetanide	Diure.	Cesamet	Nabilone	N/V

11

Brand name	Pharmacopoeal name	Main use
Ceteprin	Emepronium	Muscu.
Chendol	Chenodeoxycholate	Metab.
Chenocedon	Chenodeoxycholate	Metab.
Chloractil	Chlorpromazine	Anxio.
Chloralex	Chloral hydrate	Hypno.
Chloramate	Chlorpheniramine	Aller.
Chloramead	Chlorpromazine	Anxio.
Chlorocain	Mepivacaine	Local
Chloromide	Chlorpropamide	Diabe.
Choledyl	Choline theophyllinate	Asthm.
Chymar	Chymotrypsin	Eyes
Chymoral	Chymotrypsin	Eyes
Citanest	Prilocaine	Local
Clairvan	Ethamivan	Stimu.
Claradin	Aspirin	Analg.
Claripex	Clofibrate	Metab.
Clinazine	Trifluoperazine	Hypno.
Clinium	Lidoflazine	Arrhy.
Clinoral	Sulindac	NSAID
Clomid	Clomiphene	Hormo.
Clopixol	Zuclopenthixol	Psych.
Co-betaloc	Metoprolol	Betab.
Co-codamol	Codeine/paracetamol	Analg.
Co-codaprin	Aspirin/codeine	Analg.

Brand name	Pharmacopoeal name	Main use
Co-dydramol	Dihydrocodeine/paracetamol	Analg.
Co-proxamol	Dextropropoxyphene/paracetamol	Analg.
Cobutolin	Salbutamol	Asthm.
Codelsol	Prednisolone	Stero.
Cogentin	Benztropine	Parki.
Colofac	Mebeverine	Gut
Compazine	Prochlorperazine	N/V
Concordin	Protryptiline	Psych.
Contac	Phenylephrine	Aller.
Cordarone	Amiodarone	Arrhy.
Cordilox	Verapamil	Arrhy.
Corgard	Nadolol	Hypot.
Coro-nitro	Glyceryl trinitrate	Arrhy.
Coronex	Isosorbide dinitrate	Arrhy.
Corophyllin	Aminophylline	Asthm.
Cortelan	Cortisone	Stero.
Cortistab	Cortisone	Stero.
Cortisyl	Cortisone	Stero.
Cortogen	Cortisone	Stero.
Crystodigin	Digitoxin	Arrhy.
Cuprimine	Penicillamine	Arthr.
Cyantin	Nitrofurantoin	Antib.
Cyclimorph	Morphine/cyclizine	Analg.

Brand name	Pharmacopoeal name	Main use	Brand name	Pharmacopoeal name	Main use
Cyclobral	Cyclandelate	Vascu.	Dendrid	Idoxuridine	Micro.
Cyclogest	Progesterone	Hormo.	Depen	Penicillamine	Arthr.
Cyclokapron	Tranexamic acid	Haema.	Depixol	Flupenthixol	Psych.
Cyclospasmol	Cyclandelate	Vascu.	Depo-medrone	Methylprednisolone	Stero.
Cytacon	Cyanocobalamin	Vitam.	Deponit	Glyceryl trinitrate	Arrhy.
Cytamen	Cyanocobalamin	Vitam.	Deseril	Methisergide	Epile.
Cytoxan	Cyclophosphamide	Neopl.	Deseril	Methysergide	Migra.
Daktarin	Miconazole	Antib.	Desferal	Desferrioxamine	Iron
Dalmane	Flurazepam	Hypno.	Desoxyn	Methamphetamine	Stimu.
Daneral	Pheniramine	Hista.	Dexedrine	Dexamphetamine	Stimu.
Dantoin	Phenytoin	Epile.	DF118	Dihydrocodeine	Analg.
Dantrium	Dantrolene	Muscu.	Diabenese	Chlorpropamide	Diabe.
Daonil	Glibenclamide	Diabe.	Diamicron	Glicazide	Diabe.
Darvon	Propoxyphene	Analg.	Diamox	Acetazolamide	Diure.
DDAVP	Desmopressin	Metab.	Diatensec	Spironolactone	Diure.
Debendox	Dicyclomine	Muscu.	Diatuss	Pholcodine	Respi.
Decadron	Dexamethasone	Stero.	Diazemuls	Diazepam	Anxio.
Decaserpyl	Reserpine	Hypot.	Diazemuls	Valium	Anxio.
Declinax	Debrisoquine	Hypot.	Diazide	Triamterene	Diure.
Decortisyl	Prednisolone	Stero.	Dibenyline	Phenoxybenzamine	Hypot.
Defencin	Isoxsuprine	Vascu.	Dibucaine	Nupercaine	Local
Deltasone	Prednisolone	Stero.	Diconal	Dipipanone	Narco.
Deltastab	Prednisolone	Stero.	Dicynene	Ethamsylate	Haema.
Demerol	Pethidine	Analg.	Difflam	Benzydamine	Analg.

11

Brand name	Pharmacopoeal name	Main use	Brand name	Pharmacopoeal name	Main use
Dihydergot	Dihydroergotamine	Migra.	Dozine	Chlorpromazine	Anxio.
Dilantin	Phenytoin	Epile.	Dramamine	Dimenhydrinate	Hista.
Dimelor	Acetohexamide	Diabe.	Droleptan	Droperidol	Anxio.
Dimotane	Brompheniramine	Hista.	Dromoran	Levorphanol	Analg.
Dindevan	Phenindione	Haema.	Dryptal	Frusemide	Diure.
Diprosone	Betamethasone	Stero.	Dulcolax	Bisacodyl	Laxat.
Dirythmin	Disopyramide	Arrhy.	Duogastrone	Carbenoxalone	Gastr.
Disipal	Orphenadrine	Parki.	Duphalac	Lactulose	Gut
Disprol	Paracetamol	Analg.	Duphaston	Dydrogesterone	Hormo.
Distalgaesic	Dextropropoxephene	Analg.	Durabolin	Nandrolone	Hormo.
Distamine	Penicillamine	Arthr.	Duranest	Etidocaine	Local.
Diumide	Frusemide	Diure.	Duromine	Phentermine	Metab.
Diurexan	Xipamide	Diure.	Duromorph	Morphine	Analg.
Diuril	Chlorthiazide	Diure.	Duvalidan	Isoxsuprine	Vascu.
Dixarit	Clonidine	Hypot.	Dyazide	Triamterene/thiazide	Diure.
Dobutrex	Dobutamine	Arrhy.	Dyrenium	Triamterene	Diure.
Dolobid	Diflunisal	Analg.	Dytac	Triamterene	Diure.
Doloxene	Dextropropoxyphene	Analg.	Dytide	Triamterene/thiazide	Diure.
Domical	Amitriptyline	Psych.	Eaca	Aminocaproic acid	Haema.
Dopamet	Methyl dopa	Hypot.	Edecrin	Ethacrynic acid	Diure.
Dopram	Doxapram	Stimu.	Efcortelan	Hydrocortisone	Stero.
Doriden	Glutethamide	Hypno.	Effergot	Ergotamine	Migra.
Doryl	Carbachol	Choli.	Elantan	Isosorbide mononitrate	Arrhy.
Dozic	Haloperidol	Anxio.	Elavil	Amitriptyline	Psych.

Brand name	Pharmacopoeal name	Main use
Eldepryl	Selegiline	Parki.
Eltroxin	Thyroxine	Thyro.
Emeside	Ethosuxamide	Epile.
Emtexate	Methotrexate	Neopl.
Epanutin	Phenytoin	Epile.
Ephynal	Alphatocopheryl	Vitam.
Epifrin	Adrenaline	Glauc.
Epilim	Sodium valproate	Epile.
Epinephrine	Adrenaline	Arrhy.
Epodyl	Ethoglucid	Neopl.
Eppy	Adrenaline	Glauc.
Epsicapron	Aminocaproic acid	Haema.
Equanil	Meprobamate	Hypno.
Eradacin	Acrosoxacin	Micro.
Eraldin	Practolol	Betab.
Ergotrate	Ergometrine	Muscu.
Esbatal	Bethanidine	Hypot.
Esidrex	Hydrochlorthiazide	Diure.
Eskabarb	Phenobarbitone	Epile.
Estracyt	Estramustine	Neopl.
Ethrane	Enflurane	Anaes.
Etophylate	Acepifylline	Asthm.
Eudemine	Diazoxide	Hypot.
Euglucon	Glibenclamide	Diabe.

Brand name	Pharmacopoeal name	Main use
Euhypnos	Temazepam	Hypno.
Eulissin	Decamethonium	Anaes.
Eumydrin	Atropine methonitrate	Eyes
Eutonyl	Pargyline	MAOI
Evadyne	Butriptyline	Psych.
Evadyne	Butripyline	Psych.
Evoxin	Domperidone	N/V
Exirel	Pirbuterol	Asthm.
F Cortef	Fludrocortisone	Stero.
Fabahistin	Mebhydrolin	Hista.
Fabrol	Acetylcysteine	Resp.
Farlutal	Medroxyprogesterone	Hormo.
Fasigyn	Tinidazole	Micro.
Fazadon	Fazadinium	Anaes
Feldene	Piroxicam	NSAID
Femergin	Ergotamine tartrate	Migra.
Fenbid	Ibuprofen	NSAID
Fenopron	Fenoprofen	NSAID
Fentazin	Perphenazine	N/V
Flagyl	Metronidazole	Antib.
Flaxedil	Gallamine	Anaes.
Flexon	Orphenadrine	Parki.
Flolan	Prostacyclin	Metab.
Florinef	Fludrocortisone	Stero.

11

Brand name	Pharmacopoeal name	Main use
Fluothane	Halothane	Anaes.
Folvite	Folic acid	Vitam.
Famac	Salicylic Acid	NSAID
Fortagaesic	Pentazocine + paracetamol	Analg.
Fortral	Pentazocine	Analg.
Fortunam	Haloperidol	Anxio.
Franol	Ephedrine	Stimu.
Frisium	Clobazam	Anxio.
Fruben	Flurbiprofen	NSAID
Frumil	Amiloride/frusemide	Diure.
Frusid	Frusemide	Diure.
Furadantin	Nitrofurantoin	Antib.
Furosemide	Frusemide	Diure.
Galcodine	Codeine	Analg.
Galenphol	Pholcodine	Respi.
Galpseud	Pseudoephedrine	Aller.
Gardenal	Phenobarbitone	Epile.
Gestanin	Allyloestrenol	Hormo.
Gestone	Progesterone	Hormo.
Glibenese	Glipizide	Diabe.
Glucophage	Metformin	Diabe.
Glyconon	Tolbutamide	Diabe.
Glymese	Chlorpropamide	Diabe.
Glypressin	Terlipressin	Metab.

Brand name	Pharmacopoeal name	Main use
Gondafon	Glymidine	Diabe.
Gynergan	Ergotamine tartrate	Migra.
Halcion	Triazolam	Hypno.
Haldol	Haloperidol	Anxio.
Hamarin	Allopurinol	Gout
Harmogen	Piperazine oestrone	Hormo.
Hedulin	Phenindione	Haema.
Heminevrin	Chlormethiazole	Hypno.
Hepacon	Cyanocobalamin	Vitam.
Heroin	Diamorphine	Analg.
Herpid	Idoxuridine	Micro.
Hexopal	Inositol	Vascu.
Hexopal	Nicotinic acid	Vascu.
Hismanal	Astemizole	Hista.
Histalon	Chlorpheniramine	Aller.
Histryl	Diphenylpyramine	Hista.
Honvan	Fosfestrol	Neopl.
Hyalase	Hyaluronidase	Haema.
Hydergine	Co-dergocrine	Migra.
Hydrocortone	Hydrocortisone	Stero.
Hydromet	Methyl dopa/thiazide	Hypot.
Hydrosaluric	Hydrochlorthiazide	Diure.
Hygroton	Chlorthalidone	Hypot.
Hyperstat	Diazoxide	Hypot.

Brand name	Pharmacopoeal name	Main use
Hypnomidate	Etomidate	Anaes.
Hypnoval	Midazolam	Anxio.
Hypon	Aspirin/caffeine/codeine	Analg.
Hypovase	Prazosin	Hypot.
Hyprenan	Prenalterol	Arrhy.
Hyzazyme	Hyaluronidase	Haema.
Idoxene	Idoxuridine	Micro.
Iliadin	Oxymetazoline	Hista.
Imbriiol	Indomethacin	NSAID
Imferon	Iron dextran	Iron
Imodium	Loperamide	Gut
Imuran	Azathioprine	Neopl.
Inapsine	Droperidol	Anxio.
Inderal	Propanolol	Betab.
Indocid	Indomethacin	NSAID
Indolar	Indomethacin	NSAID
Indon	Phenindione	Haema.
Innovace	Enalapril	Psych.
Innovar	Droperidol/fentanyl	Anaes.
Intal	Sodium cromoglycate	Asthm.
Integrin	Oxypertine	Anxio.
Intraval	Thiopentone	Anaes.
Intron	Interferon	Neopl.
Intropin	Dopamine	Arrhy.

Brand name	Pharmacopoeal name	Main use
Inversine	Mecamylamine	Hypot.
Ionamin	Phentermine	Metab.
Ismelin	Guanethidine	Hypot.
Isobarb	Pentobarbitone	Hypno.
Isobec	Amylobarbitone	Hypno.
Isofedrol	Ephedrine	Stimu.
Isoket	Isosorbide dinitrate	Arrhy.
Isoproterenol	Isoprenaline	Arrhy.
Isoptin	Verapamil	Arrhy.
Isordil	Isosorbide	Arrhy.
Isuprel	Isoprenaline	Arrhy.
Jectofer	Iron sorbitol	Iron
Kabikinase	Streptokinase	Haema.
Kalspare	Triamterene/chlorthalidone	Diuré.
Kalten	Atenolol/amiloride	Betab.
Kemadrin	Procyclidine	Muscu.
Kenolog	Triamcinolone	Stero.
Kerecid	Idoxuridine	Micro.
Kerlone	Betaxolol	Betab.
Ketalar	Ketamine	Anaes.
Ketovite	Acetomenaphthone	Vitam.
Kiditard	Quinidine	Arrhy.
Kinidin	Quinidine	Arrhy.
Konakion	Phytomenandione	Vitam.

11

Brand name	Pharmacopoeal name	Main use
Konakion	Vitamin K	Vitam.
Korostatin	Nystatin	Antib.
Labophylline	Theophylline	Asthm.
Labrocol	Labetalol	Betab.
Lanitop	Medigoxin	Arrhy.
Lanoxin	Digoxin	Arrhy.
Lanvis	Thioguanine	Neopl.
Laracor	Oxprenolol	Betab.
Laraflex	Naproxen	NSAID
Larapam	Piroxicam	NSAID
Largactil	Chlorpromazine	Anxio.
Larodopa	Levodopa	Parki.
Lasix	Frusemide	Diure.
Lasma	Theophylline	Asthm.
Ledercort	Triamcinolone	Stero.
Lederfen	Fenbufen	NSAID
Ledermycin	Demeclocycline	Metab.
Lentizol	Amitriptyline	Psych.
Lergoban	Diphenylpyraline	Hista.
Lethidrone	Nalorphine	Stimu.
Lecovorin	Calcium folinate	Vitam.
Leukeran	Chlorambucil	Neopl.
Levarterenol	Noradrenaline	Arrhy.
Levius	Aspirin	Analg.

Brand name	Pharmacopoeal name	Main use
Levophed	Noradrenaline	Arrhy.
Lexotan	Bromazepam	Anxio.
Lexpec	Folic acid	Vitam.
Libanil	Glibenclamide	Diabe.
Libraxin	Chlordiazepoxide	Anxio.
Librium	Chlordiazepoxide	Anxio.
Lidocaine	Lignocaine	Local
Limbritol	Amitriptyline	Psych.
Lingraine	Ergotamine	Migra.
Lioresal	Baclofen	Muscu.
Liskonum	Lithium	Psych.
Litarex	Lithium	Psych.
Lodine	Etodolac	NSAID
Lomotil	Diphenoxylate + atropine	N/V
Lopid	Gemfibrozil	Metab.
Lopressor	Metoprolol	Betab.
Lopurin	Allopurinol	Gout
Lorfan	Levallorphan	Stimu.
Luminal	Phenobarbitone	Hypno.
Macrodantin	Nitrofurantoin	Antib.
Madopar	Benserazide	Parki.
Madopar	Levodopa/benserazide	Parki.
Maladrin	Ephedrine	Stimu.
Malinal	Almasilate	Gastr.

Brand name	Pharmacopoeal name	Main use
Malix	Glibenclamide	Diabe.
Marcain	Bupivicaine	Local
Marevan	Warfarin	Haema.
Marezine	Cyclizine	N/V
Marplan	Isocarboxazid	MAOI
Marsilid	Iproniazid	MAOI
Matrex	Methotrexate	Neopl.
Maxalon	Metoclopramide	N/V
Medomet	Methyl dopa	Hypot.
Medrone	Methylprednisolone	Stero.
Melitase	Chlorpropamide	Diabe.
Melleril	Thioridazine	Psych.
Menandione	Vitamin K	Vitam.
Meperidine	Pethidine	Analg.
Mephine	Mephentermine	Hypot.
Meprate	Meprobamate	Hypno.
Meptid	Meptazinol	Analg.
Meravil	Amitriptyline	Psych.
Merbentyl	Dicyclomine	Muscu.
Mestinon	Pyridostigmine	Muscu.
Mesylate	Phentolamine	Hypot.
Metaproteren	Orciprenaline	Asthm.
Metenix	Metolazone	Diure.
Methadrine	Methyl-amphetamine	Stimu.

Brand name	Pharmacopoeal name	Main use
Metramid	Metoclopramide	N/V
Mexitil	Mexilitine	Arrhy.
Mictral	Nalidixic acid	Micro.
Midamor	Amiloride	Diure.
Midrid	Isometheptene	Migra.
Midrilate	Cyclopentolate	Eyes
Migraleve	Buclizine	Migra.
Migril	Ergotamine tartrate	Migra.
Miltown	Meprobamate	Hypno.
Miochol	Acetylcholine	Eyes
Mistostat	Carbachol	Choli.
Mithracin	Plicamycin	Neopl.
Mobenol	Tolbutamide	Diabe.
Mobilan	Indomethacin	NSAID
Modecate	Fluphenazine	Psych.
Moditen	Fluphenazine	Psych.
Modrasone	Alclometasone	Stero.
Moducren	Amiloride	Diure.
Moduretic	Amiloride/thiazide	Diure.
Mogadon	Nitrazepam	Hypno.
Molipaxin	Trazodone	Psych.
Monistat	Miconazole	Antib.
Monit	Isosorbide mononitrate	Arrhy.
Monoparin	Heparin	Haema.

11

Brand name	Pharmacopoeal name	Main use	Brand name	Pharmacopoeal name	Main use
Monovent	Terbutaline	Respi.	Negram	Nalidixic acid	Micro.
Motilium	Domperidone	N/V	Nemasol	Aminosalicylate	NSAID
Motipress	Fluphenazine	Psych.	Nembutal	Pentobarbitone	Hypno.
Motrin	Ibuprofen	NSAID	Neomercazole	Carbimazole	Thyro.
MST	Morphine	Analg.	Neonaclex	Bendrofluazide	Diure.
Murcil	Chlordiazepoxide	Anxio.	Neoplatin	Cisplatin	Neopl.
Myambutol	Ethambutol	Micro.	Neosynephrine	Phenylephrine	Aller.
Myanesin	Mephenesin	Epile.	Nepenthe	Morphine	Analg.
Mycardol	Pentaerythritol	Arrhy.	Neulactil	Pericyazine	Psych.
Mygdalon	Metoclopramide	N/V	Nipride	Nitroprusside	Hypot.
Myleran	Busulphan	Neopl.	Nitrados	Nitrazepam	Hypno.
Mynah	Ethambutol/isoniazid	Micro.	Nitrocine	Glyceryl trinitrate	Arrhy.
Myotonine	Bethanechol	Gut	Nitrocontin	Glyceryl trinitrate	Arrhy.
Mysoline	Primidone	Epile.	Nitrolingual	Glyceryl trinitrate	Arrhy.
Nacton	Poldine	Gastr.	Nitronal	Glyceryl trinitrate	Arrhy.
Nandrolone	Durabolin	Stero.	Nivaquine	Chloroquine	Micro.
Naprosyn	Naproxen	NSAID	Nizoral	Ketoconazole	Micro.
Napsalgaesic	Dextropropoxyphene	Analg.	Nobrium	Medazepam	Anxio.
Narcan	Naloxone	Stimu.	Noctamid	Lormetazepam	Hypno.
Nardil	Phenelzine	MAOI	Noctec	Chloral Hydrate	Hypno.
Narphen	Phenazocine	Analg.	Noltam	Tamoxifen	Neopl.
Natulan	Procarbazine	Neopl.	Noludar	Methyprylone	Anxio.
Naturetin	Bendrofluazide	Diure.	Nolvadex	Tamoxifen	Neopl.
Navidrex	Cyclopenthiazide	Diure.	Norcuron	Vecuronium	Anaes.

Brand name	Pharmacopoeal name	Main use
Norflex	Orphenadrine	Parki.
Normison	Temazepam	Hypno.
Norpace	Disopyramide	Arrhy.
Norpramin	Desipramine	Psych.
Norval	Mianserin	Psych.
Novocaine	Procaine	Local
Novosemide	Frusemide	Diure.
Noxyflex	Noxythiolin	Antib.
Nozinan	Methotrimeprazine	Anxio.
Nu-seals	Aspirin	Analg.
Nubain	Nalbuphine	Analg.
Nuelin	Theophylline	Asthm.
Nupercaine	Cinchocaine	Local
Nydrazix	Isoniazid	Micro.
Nystan	Nystatin	Antib.
Oblivon	Methylpentinol	Hypno.
Olbetam	Acipimox	Metab.
Omnopon	Papaveretum	Analg.
Oncovin	Vincristine	Neopl.
One alpha	Alfacalcidol	Vitam.
Operidine	Phenoperidine	Analg.
Opilon	Thymoxamine	Vascu.
Optimax	Tryptophan	Psych.
Optimine	Azatadine	Aller.

Brand name	Pharmacopoeal name	Main use
Orabet	Metformin	Diabe.
Oradexon	Dexamethasone	Stero.
Orap	Pimozide	Psych.
Orimeten	Aminoglutethimide	Neopl.
Orudis	Ketoprofen	NSAID
Oruvail	Ketoprofen	NSAID
Ovestin	Oestriol	Hormo.
Pacitron	Tryptophan	Psych.
Palaprin forte	Aloxiprin	NSAID
Palaprin	Aspirin	Analg.
Paldesic	Paracetamol	Analg.
Palfium	Dextromoramide	Analg.
Panadol	Paracetamol	Analg.
Panheprin	Heparin	Haema.
Paracodin	Dihydrocodine	Analg.
Paraplatin	Carboplatin	Neopl.
Parasal	Aminosalicylic acid	NSAID
Parest	Methaqualone	Hypno.
Parfenac	Bufexamac	NSAID
Parlodel	Bromocriptine	Parki.
Parmid	Metoclopramide	N/V
Parnate	Tranylcypromine	MAOI
Paroven	Oxerutins	Haema.
Parvolex	Acetylcysteine	Resp.

11

Brand name	Pharmacopoeal name	Main use
Pavulon	Pancuronium	Anaes.
Paxalgesic	Dextropropoxyphene/paracetamol	Analg.
Paxofen	Ibuprofen	NSAID
Paxolax	Bisacodyl	Laxat.
Pendramine	Penicillamine	Arthr.
Penthrane	Methoxyflurane	Anaes.
Pentothal	Thiopentone	Anaes.
Percutol	Glyceryl trinitrate	Arrhy.
Pernivit	Acetomenaphthone	Vitam.
Persantin	Dipyridamole	Vascu.
Pethilorphan	Pethidine/levallorphan	Analg.
Phanodorm	Cyclobarbitone	Hypno
Pharmorubicin	Epirubicin	Neopl.
Phenergan	Promethazine	Anxio.
Phyllocontin	Aminophylline	Asthm.
Physeptone	Methadone	Analg.
Piriton	Chlorpheniramine	Aller.
Pitocin	Oxytocin	Hormo.
Pitressin	Argipressin	Hormo.
Pitressin	Vasopressin	Vascu.
Plaquenil	Hydroxychloroquine	Arthr.
Platosin	Cisplatin	Neopl.
Ponderax	Fenfluramine	Metab.
Ponstan	Mefenamic acid	Analg.
Ponstel	Mefenamic acid	Analg.
Pontocaine	Amethocaine	Local
Pramidex	Tolbutamide	Diabe.
Praminil	Imipramine	Psych.
Praxilene	Naftidrofuryl	Vascu.
Precortisyl	Prednisolone	Stero.
Predsol	Prednisolone	Stero.
Premarin	Oestrogens	Hormo.
Priadel	Lithium	Psych.
Primolut	Norethisterone	Hormo.
Primperan	Metoclopramide	N/V
Prindalol	Phenazocine	Analg.
Priscol	Tolazoline	Vascu.
Probanthine	Propantheline	Gut
Progesic	Fenoprofen	NSAID
Proglycem	Diazoxide	Hypot.
Progynova	Oestradiol	Hormo.
Prominal	Methylphenobarbitone	Epile.
Pronestyl	Procainamide	Arrhy.
Propaderm	Beclomethasone	Stero.
Propitocaine	Prilocaine	Local
Prostigmine	Neostigmine	Anaes.
Prostin	Alprostadil	Hormo.

Brand name	Pharmacopoeal name	Main use	Brand name	Pharmacopoeal name	Main use
Proternol	Isoprenaline	Arrhy.	Robaxin	Methocarbamol	Muscu.
Prothiaden	Dothiepin	Psych.	Robinul	Glycopyrronium	Anaes.
Provera	Medroxyprogesterone	Hormo.	Rocaltrol	Calcitriol	Vitam.
Pularin	Heparin	Haema.	Roferon	Interferon	Neopl.
Pulmadil	Rimiterol	Respi.	Rohypnol	Flunitrazepam	Hypno.
Pulmicort	Budesonide	Stero.	Rolazine	Hydrallazine	Hypot.
Questran	Cholestyramine	Metab.	Ronicol	Nicotinic acid	Vascu.
Ramodar	Etodolac	NSAID	Rougoxin	Digoxin	Arrhy.
Rastinon	Tolbutamide	Diabe.	Sabidal	Choline theophyllinate	Asthm.
Refolinon	Calcium folinate	Vitam.	Salazopyrin	Sulphasalazine	Antib.
Refolinon	Folinic acid	Vitam.	Salbulin	Salbutamol	Asthm.
Regitine	Phentolamine	Hypot.	Saluric	Chlorthiazide	Diure.
Reglan	Metoclopramide	N/V	Salzone	Paracetamol	Analg.
Reposans	Chlordiazepoxide	Anxio.	Sandimmun	Cyclosporin	Neopl.
Restoril	Temazepam	Hypno	Sanomigran	Pizotifen	Epile.
Rheumox	Azapropazone	NSAID	Sanomigran	Pizotifen	Epile.
Rhinocort	Budesonide	Stero.	Saventrine	Isoprenaline	Arrhy.
Rhumalgan	Diclofenac	NSAID	Scoline	Suxamethonium	Anaes.
Rhythmodan	Disopyramide	Arrhy.	Scopolamine	Hyoscine	N/V
Ridaura	Auranofin	Arthr	Seconal	Quinalbarbitone	Hypno.
Rifapen	Alfentanil	Narco.	Sectral	Acebutolol	Betab.
Rimafon	Isoniazid	Micro.	Securon	Verapamil	Arrhy.
Ritalin	Methylphenidate	Muscu.	Seminal	Phenobarbitone/theobromine	Hypno.
Rivotril	Clonazepam	Epile.	Serax	Oxazepam	Anxio.

11

Brand name	Pharmacopoeal name	Main use	Brand name	Pharmacopoeal name	Main use
Serc	Betahistine	N/V	Spasmonal	Alverine	Muscu.
Serenace	Haloperidol	Anxio.	Spiroctan	Spironolactone	Diure.
Serenid	Oxazepam	Anxio.	Stabinol	Chlorpropamide	Diabe.
Serophene	Clomiphene	Hormo.	Stelazine	Trifluoperazine	N/V
Serpasil	Reserpine	Hypot.	Stemetil	Prochlorperazine	N/V
Silbephylline	Diprophylline	Asthm.	Stesolid	Diazepam	Anxio.
Simplene	Adrenaline	Glauc.	Streptase	Streptokinase	Haema.
Sinemet	Carbidopa	Parki.	Stromba	Stanozolol	Stero.
Sinemet	Levodopa	Parki.	Strophanthin G	Ouabaine	Arrhy.
Sinemet	Levodopa/carbidopa	Parki.	Stugeron	Cinnarizine	N/V
Sinequan	Doxepin	Psych.	Sublimase	Fentanyl	Analg.
Sinthrome	Nicoumalone	Haema.	Sudafed	Pseudoephedrine	Aller.
Sintisone	Prednisolone	Stero.	Sulphasalazine	Salazopyrin	Antib.
Sodium Amytal	Sodium amylobarbitone	Hypno.	Surem	Nitrazepam	Hypno.
Solprin	Aspirin	Analg.	Surgam	Tiaprofenic	NSAID
Solumedrone	Methylprednisolone	Stero.	Surmontil	Trimipramine	Psych.
Somnite	Nitrazepam	Hypno.	Suscard	Glyceryl trinitrate	Arrhy.
Sommos	Chloral hydrate	Hypno.	Sustac	Glyceryl trinitrate	Arrhy.
Soneryl	Butobarbitone	Hypno.	Symcurin	Decamethonium	Anaes.
Sonislo	Isosorbide	Arrhy.	Symmetril	Amantadine	Parki.
Sorbid	Isosorbide	Arrhy.	Synacthen	Tetracosactrin	Hormo.
Sorbitrate	Isosorbide	Arrhy.	Synadrin	Prenylamine	Arrhy.
Sotacor	Sotalol	Betab.	Syndol	Paracetamol/codeine/doxylamine	Analg.
Sparine	Promazine	Anxio.			

Brand name	Pharmacopoeal name	Main use	Brand name	Pharmacopoeal name	Main use
Synkavit	Menadiol	Vitam.	Tetracaine	Amethocaine	Local
Synkavit	Menandiol	Vitam.	Thalamonal	Droperidol/fentanyl	Anaes.
Syntocinon	Oxytocin	Hormo.	Thalazole	Phthalylsulphathiazole	Antib.
Syntopressin	Lypressin	Metab.	Theodrox	Aminophylline	Asthm.
Tachostyptan	Thromboplastin	Haema.	Theograd	Theophylline	Asthm.
Tachyrol	Dihydrotachysterol	Vitam.	Thephorin	Phenindamine	Hista.
Tacrine	Tetrahydroaminoacridine	Anaes.	Thorazine	Chlorpromazine	Anxio.
Tagamet	Cimetidine	Gastr.	Tildiem	Diltiazem	Arrhy.
Talwin	Pentazocine	Analg.	Timoptol	Timolol	Glauc.
Tambocor	Flecanide	Arrhy.	Tinset	Oxatomide	Hista.
Tamofen	Tamoxifen	Neopl.	Tofranil	Imipramine	Psych.
Tavegil	Clemastine	Hista.	Tolanase	Tolazamide	Diab.
Tedral	Theophylline/ephedrine	Asthm.	Tolectin	Tolmetin	Arthr.
Tegretol	Carbamazepine	Epile.	Tolerzide	Sotalol/thiazide	Betab.
Teldrin	Chlorpheniramine	Aller.	Tolserol	Mephenesin	Muscu.
Temaril	Trimeprazine	Anxio.	Tonocard	Tocainide	Arrhy.
Tamgesic	Buprenorphine	Narco.	Torecan	Thiethylperazine	N/V
Tenavoid	Meprobamate	Hypno.	Tracrium	Atracurium	Anaes.
Tenoretic	Atenolol/chlorthalidone	Betab.	Trancopal	Chlormezanone	Anxio.
Tenormin	Atenolol	Betab.	Trandate	Labetolol	Betab.
Tensilon	Edrephonium	Muscu.	Tranmep	Meprobamate	Hypno.
Tenuate dospan	Diethylproprion	Metab.	Transiderm-nitro	Glyceryl trinitrate	Arrhy.
Terolin	Terodiline	Muscu.	Tranxene	Clorazepate	Anxio.
Tertroxin	Liothyronine	Metab.	Trasicor	Oxprenolol	Betab.

11

Brand name	Pharmacopoeal name	Main use	Brand name	Pharmacopoeal name	Main use
Trasylol	Aprotinin	Haema.	Urizide	Bendrofluazide	Diure.
Tremonil	Methixene	Parki.	Urolucosil	Sulphamethazole	Antib.
Trental	Oxpentifylline	Asthm.	Uromide	Sulphacarbamide	Antib.
Trichloryl	Triclofos	Hypno.	Urozide	Hydrochlorthiazide	Diure.
Tridil	Glyceryl trinitrate	Arrhy.	Utovlan	Norethisterone	Hormo.
Tridione	Troxidone	Epile.	Valium	Diazepam	Anxio.
Triflurin	Trifluoperazine	N/V	Vallergan	Trimeprazine	Hypno.
Triiodothyronine	Liothyronine	Metab.	Valoid	Cyclizine	N/V
Trilafon	Perphenazine	N/V	Varidase	Streptokinase	Haema.
Trilene	Trichlorethylene	Anaes.	Vascardin	Isosorbide	Arrhy.
Triludan	Terfenadine	Hista.	Vasculit	Bamethan	Vascu.
Triptafen	Amitriptyline	Psych.	Vasoxine	Methoxamine	Hypot.
Trypizol	Amitriptyline	Psych.	Vasoxyl	Methoxamine	Hypot.
Tubarine	Tubocurarine	Anaes.	Vatensol	Guanoclor	Hypot.
Tuinal	Amylobarbitone	Hypno.	Veganin	Aspirin/paracetamol/codeine	Analg.
Tuinal	Quinal + amylobarbitone	Hypno.	Velbe	Vinblastin	Neopl.
Ubretid	Distigmine	Muscu.	Ventolin	Salbutamol	Asthm.
Ukidan	Urokinase	Haema.	Vepesid	Etoposide	Neopl.
Unigesid	Paracetamol	Analg.	Veractil	Methotrimeprazine	Anxio.
Uniphyllin	Theophylline	Asthm.	Veriloid	Veratrum	Hypot.
Uridon	Chlorthalidone	Hypot.	Vertigon	Prochlorperazine	N/V
Urisal	Sodium citrate	Haema.	Viskaldix	Pindolol/clopamide	Betab.
Urispas	Flavoxate	Muscu.	Visken	Pindolol	Betab.
Uritol	Frusemide	Diure.	Vistaril	Hydroxyzine	Anxio.

Brand name	Pharmacopoeal name	Main use
Vivol	Diazepam	Anxio.
Voltarol	Diclofenac	NSAID
Welldorm	Dichlorphenazone	Hypno.
Wellferon	Interferon	Neopl.
Wyamine	Mephentermine	Hypot.
Xanax	Alprazolam	Psych.
Xseb	Salicylic acid	NSAID
Xylocaine	Lignocaine	Local

Brand name	Pharmacopoeal name	Main use
Zaditen	Ketotifen	Asthm.
Zantac	Ranitidine	Gastr.
Zarontin	Ethosuximide	Epile.
Zetran	Chlordiazepoxide	Anxio.
Zinamide	Pyrazinamide	Antib.
Zoladex	Goserelin	Neopl.
Zovirax	Acyclovir	Micro.
Zyloric	Allopurinol	Gout

Key

Alcoh.	Drugs used in alcoholism
Aller.	Anti-allergy drugs (not antihistamines)
Anaes.	Anaesthetic drugs
Analg.	Analgesic drugs (not narcotics)
Antib.	Antibiotic drugs
Anxio.	Anxiolytic drugs
Arrhy.	Anti-arrhythmic or angina drugs
Arthr.	Anti-arthritic drugs
Asthm.	Drugs used in asthma
Betab.	Beta blocker drugs
Choli.	Anticholinergic drugs
Diabe.	Antidiabetic drugs
Diure.	Diuretic drugs
Epile.	Anti-epileptic drugs
Eyes	Drugs used in ophthalmology
Gastr.	Antacid or similar type drugs
Glauc.	Drugs used for glaucoma
Gout	Antigout drugs
Gut	Drugs acting on the intestinal tract
Haema.	Drugs acting on the haematological system
Hista.	Antihistamine drugs
Hormo.	Hormone drugs

11

Key (Continued)

Hypno.	Sleep inducing drugs
Hypot.	Hypotensive drugs
Iron	Drugs for treating iron imbalance
Laxat.	Laxative drugs
Local	Local anaesthetic drugs
MAOI	Monoamine oxidase inhibitor drugs
Metab.	Drugs acting on the metabolic system
Micro.	Antimicrobial drugs
Migra.	Antimigraine drugs
Muscu.	Musculo-skeletal or arthritic drugs
Narco.	Narcotic drugs
Neopl.	Antineoplastic drugs
NSAID	Non-steroidal anti-inflammatory drugs
N/V	Drugs counteracting nausea or vomiting
Paget.	Drugs for treating Paget's disease
Parki.	Antiparkinsonian drugs
Psych.	Antidepressant drugs (not MAOI)
Resp.	Respiratory system drugs (not bronchodilators)
Stero.	Steroid drugs
Stimu.	Cerebral stimulant drugs
Thyro.	Drugs acting on the thyroid
Vascu.	Vascular system or vasodilator drugs
Vitam.	Vitamins

11.4 Drug interactions

'Drug 1' and 'Drug 2' are the columns containing the two drugs to
be mixed. Column 3 shows the effect of mixing these drugs. It is
important to look for the drug under its name and its group, e.g.
Propanolol and Beta blockers.

Drug 1	Drug 2	Effect
Acetohexamide	Phenylbutazone	Hypoglycaemia
Acyclovir	Probenecid	Increased acyclovir concentration
Alcohol	Antihypertensive	Hypotension
	Barbiturates	Potentiation of barbiturates
	General anaesthetics	Potentiation of general anaesthetics
	Phenothiazines	Potentiation of phenothiazines
Allopurinol	6-Mercaptopurine	Increased cytotoxic effects
	Azathioprine	Increased cytotoxic effects
Amiloride	Carbenoxalone.	Inhibition ulcer healing
Aminoglycosides	Anticholinesterase	Antagonism of anti-cholinesterase
	Cisplatin	Increased nephrotoxicity
Amiodarone	Digoxin	Potentiation digoxin
	Diltiazem	Increased myocardial depression
	Diuretics	More toxic with hypokaleamia
	Verapamil	Increased myocardial depression
Amphetamines	Antihypertensives	Reversal of antihyper-tensive effect
	Barbiturates	Altered CNS effects
	Ganglion blockers	Reversal of hypotension
	MAOI	Hypertensive crises
Anabolic steroids	Anticoagulants	Increased anticoagulant effect
Anaesthetics	Guanethidine	Hypotension
	Methyl dopa	Hypotension
	Reserpine	Hypotension
Analeptics	MAOI	CNS stimulation
Antacids	Sucralfate	Reduced effect
Antiarrhythmics	Any combination of two	Increased myocardial depression
Anticholinesterase	Aminoglycosides	Antagonism of anticholin-esterase
	Propanolol	Antagonism of anticholin-esterase
	Curareform relaxants	Reversal of relaxants
Anticoagulants	'Mycin' antibiotics	Potentiation of anticoagulants
	Anabolic steroids	Increased anticoagulant effect
	Barbiturates	Potentiation of barbiturates

11

Drug 1	Drug 2	Effect
Anticoagulants (cont.)	Barbiturates	Reduced anticoagulant effect
	Chloral hydrate	Increased anticoagulant effect
	Clofibrate	Increased anticoagulant effect
	Salicylates	Increased anticoagulant effect
	Tolbutamide	Hypoglycaemia
	Vitamin K	Reduced anticoagulant effect
Antihypertensives	Alcohol	Hypotension
	Amphetamines	Reversal of antihypertensive effect
	Ganglion blockers	Increased hypotension
	NSAID	Reduced antihypertensive effect
	Psychotropics	Hypotension
	Steroids	Reduced antihypertensive effect
Antiparkinsonian drugs	MAOI	CNS stimulation
Antithyroid drugs	Benzodiazepines	Increased antithyroid effect
Aspirin	Methotrexate	Increased toxicity of methotrexate
	Spirolonactone	Antagonism of diuretic
Azathioprine	Allopurinol	Increased cytotoxic effects
Barbiturates	Alcohol	Potentiation of barbiturates
	Amphetamines	Altered CNS effects
	Anticoagulants	Reduced anticoagulant effect
	Contraceptives	Reduced contraceptive reliability
	Griseofulvin	Reduced antibiotic effect
	Ketamine	Chemically incompatible
	Quinidine	Quinidine action reduced
	Steroids	Hyposteroid crisis in dependent patients
	Suxamethonium	Reduced effect of suxamethonium
Benzodiazepines	Antithyroid drugs	Increased antithyroid effect
Beta blockers	Verapamil	Asystole hypotension
	Cimetidine	Increased concentration of blocker
	Cyclopropane	Potentiation of cyclopropane
	Diltiazem	Bradycardia
	Ergotamine	Vasoconstriction
	Ketamine	Potentiation of ketamine
	Lignocaine type drugs	Bradycardia
Bilirubin	Pyrazolones	Raised bilirubin
	Salicylates	Raised bilirubin
	Sulphonamides	Raised bilirubin
Caffeine	Hypnotics	Hypnosis antagonized
Calcium	Digoxin	Enhanced dysrhythmias
Carbemazepine	Thyroxine	Increased requirements of thyroxine
Carbenoxalone	Amiloride	Inhibition of ulcer healing

Drug 1	Drug 2	Effect
Carbenoxalone	Digoxin	Increased toxicity of digoxin
	Spirolonactone	Inhibition of ulcer healing
Catecholamines	Tricyclic antidepressants	Hypertension
	Halothane	Dysrhythmias
Cephalosporins	Probenecid	Raised levels of cephalo-sporins
Chloral hydrate	Anticoagulants	Increased anticoagulant effect
Chloramphenicol	Phenytoin	Increased phenytoin levels
Cholestyramine	Digoxin	Reduced absorption of digoxin
	Thiazides	Reduced absorption thiazide
Cimetidine	Beta blockers	Increased concentration of blocker
	Flecanide	Increased concentration of flecanide
	Rifampicin	Reduced concentration of cim-etidine
Cisplatin	Aminoglycosides	Increased nephrotoxicity
Clofibrate	Anticoagulants	Increased anticoagulant effect
CNS depressants	CNS depressants	Enhanced depression, drowsiness
Contraceptives	Barbiturates	Reduced contraceptive reliability
	Phenytoin	Reduced contraceptive reliability
Corticosteroids	Phenytoin	Corticosteroid effect reduced
Curareform relaxants	Anticholinesterases	Reversal of relaxants
	Halothane	Increased hypotension
	Mycin antibiotics	Potentiation of relaxants
	Thiazides	Prolonged relaxation
Cyclopropane	Beta blockers	Potentiation of cyclopropane
Cytotoxics	Suxamethonium	Prolonged apnoea
Digoxin	Amiodorone	Potentiation of digoxin
	Antiarrhythmics	Potentiation of digoxin
	Calcium	Enhanced dysrhythmias
	Carbenoxolone	Increased toxicity of digoxin
	Cholestyramine	Reduced absorption of digoxin
	Diuretics	Potentiation of digoxin
	NSAID	Heat failure
	Propantheline	Reduced absorption due to low gut motility
	Quinine	Potentiation
	Reserpines	Bradycardia
	Suxamethonium	Enhanced digoxin toxicity
Diltiazem	Amiodorone	Increased myocardial depression
Diltiazem	Beta blockers	Bradycardia
Disulphiram	Phenytoin	Increased phenytoin levels
	Warfarin	Increased warfarin levels
Diuretic	Steroid	Antagonism of diuretic
Diuretics	Amiodarone	More toxic with hypokalaemia
	Digoxin	Potentiation of digoxin

11

Drug 1	Drug 2	Effect
Diuretics (cont.)	Flecanide	Increased toxicity with hypokalaemia
	Ganglion blockers	Potentiation of ganglion blockers
	Guanethidine	Hypotension
	MAOI	Increased hypertension
	Methyl dopa	Hypotension
	NSAID	Antagonism diuretic
	Reserpine	Hypotension
	Steroids	Hypokalaemia
	Suxamethonium	Increase in potassium
Dyflos	Suxamethonium	Potentiation of relaxant
Ecothiopate	Suxamethonium	Enhanced neuromuscular blockade
Ergotamine	Beta blockers	Vasoconstriction
Flecanide	Cimetidine	Increased concentration of flecanide
Flecanide	Diuretics	Increased toxicity with hypokalaemia
Ganglion blockers	Amphetamines	Reversal of hypotension
Ganglion blockers	Antihypertensives	Increased hypotension
Ganglion blockers	Diuretics	Potentiation of ganglion blockers
Ganglion blockers	MAOI	Hypotension
Gangloin blockers	Tricyclic antidepressant	Reversal of hypotension
General anaesthetics	Alcohol	Potentiation of general anaesthetics
Glutethamide	Steroids	Hyposteroid crisis in dependent patients
Griseofulvin	Barbiturates	Reduced antibiotic effect
Guanethidine	Anaesthetics	Hypotension
Guanethidine	Diuretics	Hypotention
Guanethidine	Sympathomimetics	Hypertension
Guanethidine	Tricyclic antidepressants	Reduced hypotensive effect
H_2 antagonists	Sucralfate	Reduced effect
Halothane	Catecholamines	Dysrhythmias
Halothane	Curareform relaxants	Increased hypotension
Halothane	Levodopa	Hypertension vasoconstriction
Heparin	Pencillin	Chemically incompatible
Heparin	Protamine	Antgonistic
Heparin	Steroids	Chemically incompatible
Hypnotics	Caffeine	Hypnosis antagonized
Indomethacin	Probenecid	Raised levels of indomethacin
Insulin	Propanolol	Hypoglycaemia
Insulin	Salicylates	Hypoglycaemia
Iron	Tetracyclines	Reduced absorption of antibiotics
Ketamine	Barbiturates	Chemically incompatible
Ketamine	Beta blockers	Potentiation of ketamine
Levodopa	Halothane	Hypertension

Drug 1	Drug 2	Effect
Lignocaine type drugs	Beta blockers	Bradycardia
MAOI	Tricyclic antidepressant	Potentiation of tricyclic
	Amphetamines	Hypertensive crises
	Analeptics	CNS stimulation
	Antiparkinsonium drugs	CNS stimulation
	Diuretics	Increased hypertension
	Ganglion blockers	Hypotension
	Opiates	Potentiation of opiates
	Phenylephrine	Potentiation of phenylephrine
	Sulphonyl ureas	Hypoglycaemia
6-Mercaptopurine	Allopurinol	Increased cytotoxic effects
Methotrexate	Aspirin	Increased toxicity of methotrexate
	NSAID	Increased toxicity of methotrexate
Methyl dopa	Anaesthetics	Hypotension
	Diuretics	Hypotension
	Sympathomimetics	Reduced hypotensive effect
	Tricyclic antidepressants	Reduced hypotensive effect
Mycin antibiotics	Anticoagulants	Potentiation of anticoagulants
	Curareform relaxants	Potentiation of relaxants
	Muscle relaxants	Potentiation of relaxation
Nalidixic acid	Probenecid	Raised levels of nalidixic acid
Naloxone	Opiate	Reversal of opiate effect
Nephrotoxic drugs	Nephrotoxic drugs	Enhancement
NSAID	Antihypertensive	Reduced effect
	Digoxin	Heart failure
	Diuretics	Antagonism of diuretic
	Methotrexate	Increased toxicity of methotrexate
Opiates	MAOI	Potentiation of opiates
	Naloxone	Reversal of opiate effect
	Pentazocine	Reduced opiate effect
PABA local anaesthetics	Sulphonamides	Reduced antibiotic effects
Penicillins	Heparin	Chemically incompatible
	Probenecid	Raised levels of penicillins
Pentazocine	Opiates	Reduced opiate effect
Phenothiazines	Alcohol	Potentiation of phenothiazines
	Ganglion blockers	Increased effect of ganglion blockers
	Steroids	Hyposteroid crisis in dependent patients
Phenylbutazone	Acetohexamide	Hypoglycaemia
	Thyroxine	False low levels of thyroxine
Phenylephrine	MAOI	Potentiation of phenylephrine
Phenytoin	Chloramphenicol	Increased phenytoin levels
	Contraceptives	Reduced contraceptive reliability
	Corticosteroids	Corticosteroid effect reduced
	Disulphiram	Increased phenytoin levels

11

Drug 1	Drug 2	Effect
Phenytoin	Pyrazolones	Potentiation of phenytoin
	Steroids	Hyposteroid crisis in dependent patients
	Sulphonamides	Potentiation of phenytoin
Physostigmine	Suxamethonium	Potentiation of relaxant
Probenecid	Cephalosporins	Raised levels of cephalosporins
	Indomethacin	Raised levels of indomethacin
	Nalidixic acid	Raised levels of nalidixic acid
	Penicillins	Raised levels of penicillins
	Salicylates	Antagonism of uricosuric effect
Procaine	Suxamethonium	Prolonged relaxation
Propanolol	Anticholinesterase	Antagonism of anticholinesterase
	Insulin	Hypoglycaemia
	Sulphonyl ureas	Hypoglycaemia
Propantheline	Digoxin	Reduced absorption due to low gut motility
Protamine	Heparin	Antagonistic
Psychotropics	Antihypertensives	Hypotension
Pyrazolones	Bilirubin	Raised bilirubin
	Phenytoin	Potentiation of phenytoin
	Sulphonyl ureas	Hypoglycaemia
Pyridostigmine	Suxamethonium	Potentiation of relaxant
Quinidine	Barbiturates	Quinidine action reduced
Quinine	Digoxin	Potentiation
Reserpine	Anaesthetics	Hypotension
	Digoxin	Bradycardia
	Diuretics	Hypotension
	Sympathomimetics	Hypertension
	Tricyclic antidepressants	Reduced hypotensive effect
Rifampicin	Cimetidine	Reduced concentration of cimetidine
Salicylates	Anticoagulants	Increased anticoagulant effect
	Bilirubin	Raised bilirubin
	Insulin	Hypoglycaemia
	Methotrexate	Increased cytotoxic effect
	Probenecid	Antagonism of uricosuric effect
	Sulphonamides	Increased antibiotic effect
	Sulphonyl ureas	Hypoglycaemia
Spirolonactone	Carbenoxalone	Inhibition of ulcer healing
	Aspirin	Antagonism of diuretic
Steroids	Antihypertensives	Reduced effect
	Barbiturates	Hyposteroid crisis in dependent patients
	Diuretics	Antagonism of diuretic Hypokalaemia

Drug 1	Drug 2	Effect
Steroids	Glutethamide	Hyposteroid crisis of dependent patients
	Heparin	Chemically incompatible
	Phenothiazines	Hyposteroid crisis in dependent patients
	Phenytoin	Hyposteroid crisis in dependent patients
	Thiazides	Hyperglycaemia
	Tricyclic antidepressants	Chemically incompatible
Sucralfate	Antacids	Reduced effect
	H$_2$ antagonists	Reduced effect
Sulphafurazole	Thiopentone	Increased effect of thiopentone
Sulphonamides	Bilirubin	Raised bilirubin
	PABA local anaesthetics	Reduced antimicrobial effect
	Phenytoin	Potentiation of phenytoin
	Salicylates	Increased antibiotic effect
	Sulphonyl ureas	Hypoglycaemia
Sulphonyl ureas	MAOI	Hypoglycaemia
	Propanolol	Hypoglycaemia
	Pyrazolones	Hypoglycaemia
	Salicylates	Hypoglycaemia
	Sulphonamides	Hypoglycaemia
Suxamethonium	Barbiturates	Reduced effect of suxamethonium
	Cytotoxics	Prolonged apnoea
	Digoxin	Enhanced digoxin toxicity
	Diuretics	Increase in potassium
	Dyflos	Potentiation of relaxants
	Ecothiopate	Enhanced neuromuscular blockade
	Physostigmine	Potentiation of relaxant
	Procaine	Prolonged relaxation
	Pyridostigmine	Potentiation of relaxant
	Trifluperazine	Reduced effect of suxamethonium
Sympathomimetics	Guanethidine	Hypertension
	Methyl dopa	Reduced hypotensive effect
	Reserpine	Hypertension
Tetracyclines	Iron	Reduced absorption of antibiotic
	Iron	Reduced absorption of antibiotics
Thiazides	Cholestyramine	Reduced absorption of thiazides
	Curareform relaxants	Prolonged relaxation
	Steroids	Hyperglycaemia
Thiopentone	Sulphafurazole	Increased effect of thiopentone
Thyroxine	Carbemazepine	Increased thyroxine requirements
	Phenylbutazone	False low thyroxine levels

11

Drug 1	Drug 2	Effect
Tolbutamide	Anticoagulants	Hypoglycaemia
Tricyclic antidepressants	Catecholamines	Hypertension
	Ganglion blocker	Reversal of hypotension
	Guanethidine	Reduced hypotensive effect
	MAOI	Potentiation of tricyclic
	Methyl dopa	Reduced hypotensive effect
	Reserpine	Reduced hypotensive effect
	Steroids	Chemically incompatible
	Vasoconstrictor	Potentiation
Trifluperazine	Suxamethonium	Reduced effect of suxa-methonium
Vasoconstrictors	Tricyclics	Potentiation of constriction
Verapamil	Amiodarone	Increased myocardial depression
	Beta blocker	Asystole hypotension
Vitamin K	Anticoagulants	Decreased anticoagulant effect
Warfarin	Disulphiram	Increased warfarin levels

Section 12
Toxicology

12.1 Introduction to toxicology

A brief guide is given to therapeutic and toxic concentrations of some common drugs and other substances (National Poisons Unit, Guv's Hospital).

Notes

1 All drug concentrations are measured in plasma except where otherwise specified.

2 All drug concentrations are expressed in units of µg/ml (equivalent to mg/l) except where otherwise stated. SI units are not used yet in poisons centres.

3 The data quoted in this guide are based on both the results obtained in this unit as well as reliable sources in the scientific literature.

4 The concentrations quoted in this guide must be regarded as only approximations, which do not take into account certain variables which may modify individual drug response, i.e. weight, other medication, etc.

5 If in any doubt, the poison centres given below (with telephone numbers) will offer any doctor immediate information and guide to treatment.

12.1.1 Poisons information services

Belfast	0232-240503
Birmingham	021-554 3801
Cardiff	0222-709901
Dublin	0001-745588
Edinburgh	031-229 2477
	031-228 2441 (Viewdata)
Leeds	0532-430715 *or* 0532-432799
London (National Poisons Information Centre)	01-635 9191 *or* 01-407 7600
Newcastle	091-232 5131

12

12.2 Drug levels and toxic levels

The values below are in mass units, i.e. mg/l, except where
marked. If your laboratory gives results in other units ask them to
convert to the mass unit to allow for interpretation.

Substance	Therapeutic/ normal range (mg/l)	Severe toxic levels greater than (mg/l)	First line antidote
Acids			
Amiodarone	1–2	4	
Amitriptyline	0.1–0.2	1	Pyridostigmine
Amphetamine	0.1–0.2	0.5	
Antidepressants			Haemoperfusion
Arsenic (blood)	<30 µg/l	50 µg/l	5 mg/kg i.m. dimercaprol
Arsenic (hair)	<1 µg/l	2 µg/l	5 mg/kg i.m. dimercaprol
Arsenic (urine)	<40 µg/l	200 µg/l	5 mg/kg i.m. dimercaprol
Aspirin	150–250	500	Forced alkaline diuresis
Barbiturates			Conservative
Amylobarbitone	2–5	40	
Barbitone	5–15	100	Forced alkaline diuresis
Butobarbitone	2–10	80	
Cyclobarbitone	2–5	40	
Heptabarbitone	2–5	40	
Hexabarbitone	2–5	40	
Pentobarbitone	2–5	40	
Phenobarbitone	5–30	100	Forced alkaline diuresis
Quinalbarbitone	2–5	40	
Beta blockers			Atropine/glucagon/ isoprenaline
Bleach			2.5% sodium thiosulphate solution
Bromide	3–4	500	
Cadmium (blood)	<10 µg/l	20 µg/l	
Cadmium (urine)	<10 µg/l	20 µg/l	
Carbamazepine	1.5–9	50	
Carbon monoxide	0.3–2%	20%	Oxygen
Chlomipramine	<0.5	1	
Chloral	5–10	80	
Chloramphenicol	10–20	40	
Chlordiazepoxide	0.5–1	10	Flumazenil 200 µg i.v.
Chlormethiazole	0.1–2	20	
Chloroquine	<0.2	1	
Chlorpromazine	0.1	1	Procyclidine/conservative
Cholinesterase inhibitors			Pralidoxime/atropine
Clonazepam	<0.05	1	Flumazenil 200 µg i.v.
Cocaine	<0.3	3	Propanolol/diazepam
Codeine	<0.10	1	0.4 mg i.v. naloxone

Substance	Therapeutic/ normal range (mg/l)	Severe toxic levels greater than (mg/l)	First line antidote
Copper	1–2	5	Penicillamine/dimercaprol
Coumarins			Vitamin K
Cyanides	0.04	1	Cobalt edetate/25% thiosulphate
Desalkylflurazepam	<0.15	2	
Desipramine	0.05–0.15	1	
Dextropropoxyphene	0.2–0.3	1	0.4 mg i.v. naloxone
Diazepam	1–2	5	Flumazenil 200 µg i.v.
Digitoxin	14–30 µg/l	30 µg/l	
Digoxin	1–2 µg/l	4 µg/l	
Dinitroorthocresol		50	
Diphenhydramine	0.1–1	5	
Disopyramide	2–3	8	
Dothiepin	<0.3	1	
Doxepin	<0.2	1	
Epanutin	10–20		
Ethambutol	3–5	6	
Ethanol		3000	Conservative
Ethchlorvynol	10–20	100	
Ethosuxamide	40–80	250	
Ethylene glycol		500	50 g ethanol oral
Fenfluramine	0.1–0.2	0.5	
Flunitrazepam	<0.05	1	Flumazenil 200 µg i.v.
Fluorides		2.5	Calcium gluconate 10 ml i.v.
Gentamicin	8–10	15	
Glutethimide	2–4	30	
Gold			Dimercaprol
Haloperidol	<0.1	0.5	Benztropine
Heparin	kcct<3	kcct>4	Protamine
Hydrogen sulphide			Sodium nitrate
Imipramine	0.1–0.3	1.0	
Indomethacin	0.7–1.3		
Iron	<1.8	5	Desferrioxamine 2 g/l solution
Isoniazid	3–10	50	
Lead	<1.4 µmol/l	>3.8	Sod-calc edetate/dimercaprol
Lignocaine	2–5	8	
Lithium	0.8–1.3 mmol/l	2	
Lorazepam	<0.20	2	Flumazenil 200 µg i.v.
Maprotiline	0.1–0.3	0.5	
Meprobamate	5–10	100	
Mercury (blood)	<15 µg/l	40	5 mg/kg i.m. dimercaprol
Mercury (urine)	<20 µg/l	100	5 mg/kg i.m. dimercaprol
Methadone	0.05–0.1	1	0.4 mg i.v. naloxone
Methanol		200	Ethanol
Methaqualone	2–4	20	
Methyprylone	10–20	30	
Methsuximide	10–40	40	
Methylamphetamine	<0.05	0.3	
Mexiletine	<1.5	3	

12

Substance	Therapeutic/ normal range (mg/l)	Severe toxic levels greater than (mg/l)	First line antidote
Mianserin	<0.1	0.5	
MAOI			Chlorpromazine
Morphine	0.05–0.1	0.3	0.4 mg i.v. naloxone
Mysolin	5–12		
Nitrazepam	<0.2	2	Flumazenil 200 µg i.v.
Nordiazepam	<1.5	5	Flumazenil 200 µg i.v.
Nortryptyline	0.05–0.15	1	
Organophosphates			1 g i.v. pralidoxime/atropine 2 mg
Orphenadrine	0.1–0.2	2	
Oxalic acid		5	1% calcium gluconate solution orally
Oxazepam	1–2	5	Flumazenil 200 µg i.v.
Oxprenolol	<0.2	2	Atropine/inotropes
Oxyphenbutazone	<100	200	
Paracetamol	20–30	200	2.5 g methionine po/acetylcysteine i.v.
Paraquat		0.5	Fullers earth
Pentazocine	<0.2	1	0.4 mg i.v. naloxone
Pethidine	0.2–0.8	2	0.4 mg i.v. naloxone
Phenacetin			25 ml 1% methylene blue
Phenothiazines			Procyclidine
Phenylbutazone	50–100	200	
Phenytoin	7–20	40	Haemoperfusion
Primidone	3–12	100	Haemoperfusion
Procainamide	4–8	16	
Propanolol	0.05–0.10	2	Atropine/inotropes
Protriptyline	0.1–0.2	1	
Quinidine	3–5	10	
Quinine	3–5	10	
Salicylate	150–250	500	Forced alkaline diuresis
Snake bite			Zagreb antivenom
Sodium valproate	50–80	200	
Sulthiame	<12	30	
Tegretol	4–12		
Thallium (blood)	<10 µg/l	100	Potassium hexacyanoferrate
Thallium (urine)	<20 µg/l	500	10 g oral (i.e. Prussian blue)
Theophylline	8–20	40	Propanolol/haemoperfusion
Thoridazine	<1	5	
Trichlorethanol	5–10	80	
Trimipramine	<0.3	1.0	
Verapamil	0.1–0.2	4.0	Symptomatic
Warfarin	1–3	10	Vitamin K
Zinc	0.7–1.5		

Where no first line antidote is given, treatment for that substance is in general supportive.

12.3 Drug overdose treatment

The current mortality from overdose is less than 3%. Respiratory complications are the principal cause of death, from respiratory depression or inhalation of vomit. The main treatment is therefore to maintain the airway and to provide cardiovascular and respiratory support while the body eliminates the poison.

Gastric emptying is considered useful in all salicylate and antidepressant overdoses ingested within 8–10 hours, and in recent ingestion of other drugs where potentially large amounts have been taken. The patient should be conscious. In the semi-conscious or unconcious patient, endotracheal intubation will be needed before gastric lavage is performed.

300 ml of water (*not* saline) at approximately 38 C is passed through a large bore tube repeatedly until clear lavage is achieved.

Other treatments for specific drug overdoses are given below.

12.3.1 Repeat activated oral charcoal

Repeated dosing with oral activated charcoal will increase the elimination of many drugs and is simpler and less invasive than other techniques. It is particularly effective in the case of
phenobarbitone;
salicylates;
theophyllines;
phenytoin;
carbamazepine.

Suggested regime
1 50–100 g activated charcoal orally or by NG tube when the patient arrives in hospital.
2 50 g 4 hourly until recovery or plasma concentration have fallen to safe levels.

12

12.3.2 Forced alkaline diuresis

This is of value only with overdoses of
salicylates
phenobarbitone
barbitone

The emphasis should be in achieving an alkaline urine rather than a massive diuresis.

Suggested regime
1 Urinary catheter, CVP line, electrolytes, blood sugar, measure blood gases.
2 500 ml 5% dextrose +1 g KCl 500 ml 1.26% sodium bicarbonate +1 g KCl 500 ml 5% dextrose +1 g KCl.
(These should be given intravenously over the first hour then repeated over the next 2 hours or so to produce a urine output of 250–500 ml/h with a pH >7.5 using 20–40 mg frusemide if necessary.)
3 Monitor electrolytes and blood gases 2 hourly (blood pH <7.6 at all times). CVP, BP, urine output, etc. should be monitored every 15 minutes.

12.3.3 Forced acid diuresis

This probably has no role nowadays and is of very limited value only with overdoses of
quinine
phencyclidine
amphetamine

Suggested regime
As above with the following fluids: 1000 ml 5% dextrose +1 g KCl 500 normal saline +1.0 g KCl +1.5 g ammonium chloride (or 10 g arginine) (if neither are available then 2 g/h oral ammonium chloride can be used).

These should be given intravenously over the first hour then repeated over the next 2 hours or so to produce a urine output of 500 ml/h with a pH <6.5 using 20–40 mg frusemide if necessary.

Monitor electrolytes and blood gases 2 hourly. CVP, BP, urine output, etc. should be monitored every 15 minutes.

12.3.4 Haemoperfusion

This may be of value with a few severe drug overdoses but should be embarked upon with great care. The technique is invasive and potentially hazardous, thus treatment should be dictated by clinical severity of poisoning as well as drug concentrations.

The plasma drug levels should be over the severe toxic levels; see p. 236 before considering this technique. It is of no use in the treatment of overdoses due to:
tricyclic antidepressants
benzodiazepines
alcohols
phenothiazines
heavy metals
snake bites
aldehydes
propoxyphenes
cyanides
All other groups may show variable benefit from treatment.

In all cases of overdose the poisons units will advise on the best treatment, so if in any doubt call them.

12

Section 13
SI Units and Conversion Tables

13

13.1 SI units

13.1.1 Basic units

In 1960 at the Conférence Générale des Poids et Mésures in France, the international units were formulated to standardize methods of denoting units and decimal points.

This was enlarged and developed into the Système International d'Unités (SI units) and came into force in the UK on 1st October 1975.

The following list gives the basic SI units and their derivations, together with their recognized abbreviations. The letters l, m, t denote the basic concept of *length, mass, time* from which the definitions of the derived units can be obtained.

For example, force can be represented as:

$$\frac{\text{mass} \times \text{length}}{\text{time}^2}$$

or mass × acceleration.

metre	m	unit of length (l)
kilogram	kg	unit of mass (m)
second	s	unit of time (t)
kelvin	K	unit of temperature
candela	cd	unit of light
decibel	db	unit of sound (1 decibel = 1/10 bel)
ampere	A	unit of electrical current $\equiv 2 \times 10^{-7}$ newton/metre
hertz	Hz	unit of frequency per second
mole	mol	unit of amount of substance in grams
newton	N	unit of force (which gives 1 kilogram mass an acceleration of 1 metre per second² (ml/t^{-2}) = joule/metre
pascal	Pa	unit of pressure (force per unit area ($ml^{-1}t^{-2}$) = 1 newton/metre²)
joule	J	unit of energy or work force through a distance (ml^2t^{-2}) = 1 newton metre
watt	W	unit of power (energy per second (ml^2t^{-3}) = 1 newton metre/second = joule/second)
coulomb	C	unit of quantity of electricity = 1 ampere second
volt	V	unit of electrical potential $= (ml^2t^{-3}A^{-1}) = \dfrac{1 \text{ watt}}{1 \text{ ampere}}$ $= \dfrac{1 \text{ joule}}{1 \text{ ampere second}}$

13

ohm   Ω   unit of electrical $= (ml^2t^{-3}A^{-2})$
              resistance

$$= \frac{1 \text{ volt}}{1 \text{ ampere}}$$

13.1.2 SI fractions or multiples

10^{18}	exa	E	10^{-18}	atto	a
10^{15}	peta	P	10^{-15}	femto	f
10^{12}	tera	T	10^{-12}	pico	p
10^{9}	giga	G	10^{-9}	nano	n
10^{6}	mega	M	10^{-6}	micro	μ
10^{3}	kilo	k(K)	10^{-3}	milli	m
10^{1}	deca	da(D)	10^{-1}	deci	d

In this book we have, where possible, used the SI units. However, since the conversion depends on knowledge of the molecular weights, certain units cannot be in SI units. In these cases they remain in the old units.

13.2 Conversion tables for physical units

13.2.1 Length

1 mm	= 0.0394 inches	1 inch (in)	= 25.4 mm
1 metre	= 1.0936 yards (yd)	1 foot (ft)	= 304.8 mm
1 km	= 0.6214 miles	1 yard (yd)	= 0.9144 m
1 ångström (Å)	$= 10^{-1}$ nanometres (nm)	1 mile	= 1.6093 km
		1 nautical mile	= 1.852 km

13.2.2 Weight

1 g	= 0.0353 oz	1 ounce (oz)	= 0.4725 grains
			= 0.02835 kg
1 kg	= 2.2046 lb	1 pound (lb)	= 0.4536 kg
1000 kg	= 0.9842 tons	1 ton	= 2240 lb = 1016.06 kg
1 mg	= 0.0167 grains	1 grain	= 64.79 mg
1 kg	= 0.1575 stones	1 stone	= 6.35 kg
1 tonne (t)	= 1000 kg	1 cwt	= 112 lb = 50.8 kg

13.2.3 Temperature

0 kelvin (K) $= -273°C$ (absolute zero)
273.15 K $= 0°C = 32°F$ $°C = (°F - 32) \times 5/9$
373.16 K $= 100°C = 212°F$ $°F = (°C \times 9/5) + 32$

°C	°F		°C	°F
30	86.0		36	96.8
31	87.8		37	98.6
32	89.6		38	100.4
33	91.4		39	102.2
34	93.2		40	104.0
35	95.0		41	105.8

13.2.4 Area

1 mm²	= 0.00155 in²	
1 m²	= 10.764 ft²	
1 m²	= 1.1960 yd²	
10 000 m²	= 1 hectare	= 2.4711 acres
1 km²	= 100 hectares	= 0.3861 miles²
4046.86 m³	= 1 acre	= 4840 yd²
1 in²	= 645.16 mm²	
1 ft²	= 144 in²	= 0.0929 m²
1 yd²	= 9 ft²	= 0.8361 m²
1 mile²	= 2.5899 km²	

13.2.5 Volume

1 litre (l)	= 1 dm³	
1000 ml	= 0.03531 ft³	
1 m³	= 1.3080 yd³	
1 l	= 0.22 gallons	
1 ml	= 16.9 minims	
1 l	= 1.76 pints	
1 ml	= 0.282 fluid drachm	
1 fluid drachm	= 3.55 ml	
1 ml	= 0.0352 fluid oz	
1 fluid oz	= 28.42 ml	
1 in³	= 16.387 cm³	
1 ft³ = 1728 in³	= 0.028317 m³ = 28.317 litres	
1 yd³ = 27 ft³	= 0.7646 m³	
1 gallon (UK)	= 4.546 l	
1 minim	= 0.0592 ml	
1 pint	= 0.5683 l	= 20 fluid oz

13

```
1 teaspoon       = 4.5 ml   ⎫
1 tablespoon     = 15 ml    ⎬ approx.
1 teacup         = 120 ml   ⎭
1 dessertspoon   = 8 ml     ⎫
1 wine glass     = 60 ml    ⎬ approx.
1 tumbler glass  = 240 ml   ⎭
```

13.2.6 Speed

1 km/h = 0.2778 m/s   1 m/s = 3.6 km/h
1 knot = 1.852 km/h = 1.6 mph
1 km/h = 0.625 mph   1 mph = 1.6 km/h

13.2.7 Pressure

1 mmHg	= 1.36 cmH_2O	= 133.3 N/m^2	= 0.0194 psi
		= 0.133 kPa	
1 cmH_2O	= 98.06 N/m^2	= 0.09806 kPa	
1 psi	= 0.070 kg/cm^2	= 51.7 mmHg	= 70.3 cmH_2O
	= 6894.76 N/m^2	= 6.895 kPa	

1 atmosphere absolute = 760 mmHg = 14.7 psi = 29.9 inHg
                      = 1.03 kg/cm^2
                      = 1.0133×10^5 N/m^2 = 101.33 kPa = 1035 cmH_2O
                      = 1 bar = 1000 millibars
1 kPa   = 0.146 psi = 1.0×10^3 N/m^2

13.2.8 Work/energy

1 joule (J)   = 1 Nm
1 J   = 10^7 ergs = 0.239 calories (cal)
1 cal   = 4.1868 J
1 BTU   = 1055 J
1 kilowatt hour (kwh) = 3.6×10^6 J

13.2.9 Power

1 watt   = 1 newton metre/second = 1 J/s
1 horse power = 746 watts = 550 foot pound/second = 746 Nm/s
1 metre kilogram/second = 9.81 watts = 9.81 Nm/s

13.2.10 Force

1 newton (N)   = 10^5 dynes
1 kilogram force (kgf) = 9.807 N
1 pound force (lbf)   = 4.44 N

13.3 Medical catheter gauge conversion table

SWG	Diameter (in)	Diameter (mm)	English gauge	French charriere
–	0.0156	0.390	–	1
26	0.018	0.457	–	–
–	0.019	0.500	00	–
25	0.020	0.508	–	–
24	0.022	0.559	–	–
23	0.024	0.610	–	–
–	0.026	0.660	–	2
22	0.028	0.711	–	–
21	0.032	0.813	–	–
20	0.036	0.914	–	–
–	0.039	1	0	3
19	0.040	1.02	–	–
18	0.048	1.22	–	–
17	0.056	1.42	–	4
–	0.059	1.50	1	–
16	0.064	1.62	–	–
–	0.066	1.66	–	5
15	0.072	1.82	–	–
–	0.079	2	2	6
14	0.080	2.03	–	–
13	0.092	2.33	–	7
–	0.098	2.50	3	–
12	0.104	2.64	–	–
–	0.105	2.66	–	8
11	0.116	2.95	–	–
–	0.118	3	4	9
10	0.128	3.25	–	–
–	0.131	3.33	–	10
–	0.138	3.50	5	–
9	0.144	3.66	–	11
–	0.157	4	6	12
8	0.160	4.06	–	–
–	0.170	4.33	–	13
7	0.176	4.47	–	–
–	0.177	4.50	7	–
–	0.183	4.66	–	14
6	0.192	4.87	–	–
–	0.197	5	8	15
–	0.210	5.33	–	16
5	0.212	5.38	–	–
–	0.217	5.50	9	–
–	0.233	5.66	–	17

13

SWG	Diameter (in)	Diameter (mm)	English gauge	French charriere
4	0.232	5.89	–	–
–	0.236	6.00	10	18
–	0.249	6.33	–	19
3	0.252	6.40	–	–
–	0.256	6.50	11	–
–	0.262	6.66	–	20
–	0.275	7	12	21
2	0.276	7.01	–	–
–	0.288	7.33	–	22
–	0.295	7.50	13	–
1	0.300	7.64	–	–
–	0.301	7.66	–	23
–	0.315	8	14	24
–	0.328	8.33	–	25
–	0.344	8.50	15	–
–	0.341	8.66	–	26
–	0.354	9	16	27
–	0.367	9.33	–	28
–	0.374	9.50	17	–
–	0.380	9.66	–	29
–	0.393	10	18	30
–	0.406	10.33	–	31
–	0.413	10.50	19	–
–	0.419	10.66	–	32
–	0.433	11	20	33
–	0.446	11.33	–	34
–	0.453	11.50	21	–
–	0.459	11.66	–	35
–	0.472	12	22	36
–	0.485	12.33	–	37
–	0.492	12.50	23	–
–	0.498	12.66	–	38
–	0.511	13	24	39

Benique gauge = 2 × French (charriere) gauge.

13.4 Surface area nomograms

13.4.1 Infants and children

Ventilation, certain drug dosages, basal metabolic rate and lean body mass are more accurately assessed from surface area than from age, weight and height, etc.

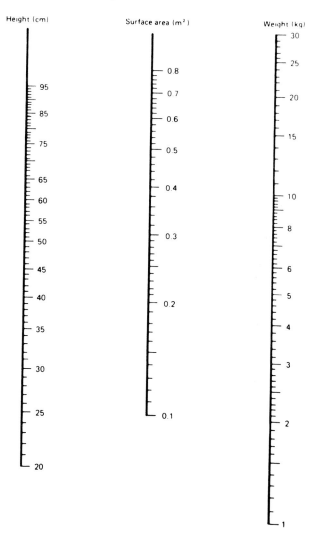

13

13.4.2 Adults

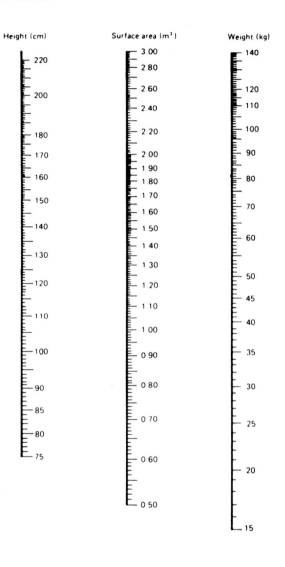

Height (cm)   Surface area (m²)   Weight (kg)

13.5 Percentile graphs

13.5.1 Paediatric age : height

This graph shows height at ages 0–10 years. The 10th, 50th and 90th percentiles shown are each an average of male and female heights.

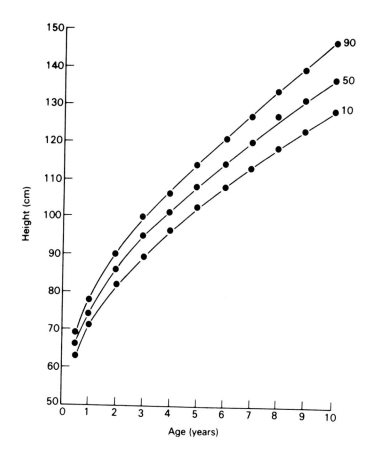

13

13.5.2 Paediatric age:weight

This graph shows weight at ages 0–10 years. The 10th, 50th and 90th percentiles shown are an average of male and female weights.

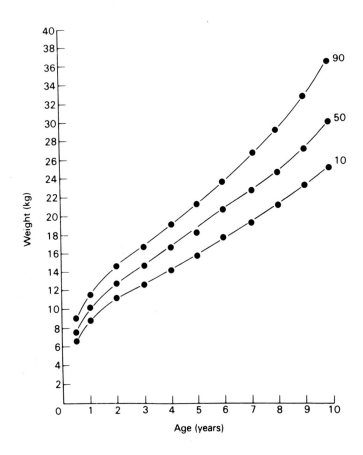

13.5.3 Desirable weights of adults according to height and frame

Height without shoes			Desirable weight in kg and pounds (in indoor clothing). ages 25 and over						
			Small frame		Medium frame		Large frame		
metres	ft	in	kg	lb	kg	lb	kg	lb	
Men									
1.550	5	1	50.8–54.4	112–120	53.5–58.5	118–129	57.2–64	126–141	
1.575	5	2	52.2–55.8	115–123	54.9–60.3	121–133	58.5–65.3	129–144	
1.600	5	3	53.5–57.2	118–126	56.2–61.7	124–136	59.9–67.1	132–148	
1.625	5	4	54.9–58.5	121–129	57.6–63	127–139	61.2–68.9	135–152	
1.650	5	5	56.2–60.3	124–133	59–64.9	130–143	62.6–70.8	138–156	
1.675	5	6	58.1–62.1	128–137	60.8–66.7	134–147	64.4–73	142–161	
1.700	5	7	59.9–64	132–141	62.6–68.9	138–152	66.7–75.3	147–166	
1.725	5	8	61.7–65.8	136–145	64.4–70.8	142–156	68.5–77.1	151–170	
1.750	5	9	63.5–68	140–150	66.2–72.6	146–160	70.3–78.9	155–174	
1.775	5	10	65.3–69.9	144–154	68–74.8	150–165	72.1–81.2	159–179	
1.800	5	11	67.1–71.7	148–158	69.9–77.1	154–170	74.4–83.5	164–184	
1.825	6	0	68.9–73.5	152–162	71.7–79.4	158–175	76.2–85.7	168–189	
1.850	6	1	70.8–75.7	156–167	73.5–81.6	162–180	78.5–88	173–194	
1.875	6	2	72.6–77.6	160–171	75.7–83.5	167–185	80.7–90.3	178–199	
1.900	6	3	74.4–79.4	164–175	78.1–86.2	172–190	82.7–92.5	182–204	

13

13.5.3 (Continued)

Desirable weight in kg and pounds (in indoor clothing), ages 25 and over

Height without shoes		Small frame		Medium frame		Large frame	
metres	ft in	kg	lb	kg	lb	kg	lb
Women							
1.425	4 8	41.7–44.5	92–98	43.5–48.5	96–107	47.2–54	104–119
1.450	4 9	42.6–45.8	94–101	44.5–49.9	98–110	48.1–55.3	106–122
1.475	4 10	43.5–47.2	96–104	45.8–51.3	101–113	49.4–56.7	109–125
1.500	4 11	44.9–48.5	99–107	47.2–52.6	104–116	50.8–58.1	112–128
1.525	5 0	46.3–49.9	102–110	48.5–54	107–119	52.2–59.4	115–131
1.550	5 1	47.6–51.3	105–113	49.9–55.3	110–122	53.5–60.8	118–134
1.575	5 2	49–52.6	108–116	51.3–57.2	113–126	54.9–62.6	121–138
1.600	5 3	50.3–54	111–119	52.6–59	116–130	56.7–64.4	125–142
1.625	5 4	51.7–55.8	114–123	54.4–61.2	120–135	58.5–66.2	129–146
1.650	5 5	53.5–57.6	118–127	56.2–63	124–139	60.3–68	133–150
1.675	5 6	55.3–59.4	122–131	58.1–64.9	128–143	62.1–69.9	137–154
1.700	5 7	57.2–61.2	126–135	59.9–66.7	132–147	64–71.7	141–158
1.725	5 8	59–63.5	130–140	61.7–68.5	136–151	65.8–73.9	145–163
1.750	5 9	60.8–65.3	134–144	63.5–70.3	140–155	67.6–76.2	149–168
1.775	5 10	62.6–67.1	138–148	65.3–72.1	144–159	69.4–79	153–174

Index